The Trans Fat Free Kitchen

THE
Trans Fat Free
KITCHEN

SIMPLE RECIPES • SHOPPING GUIDES
RESTAURANT TIPS

Ronni Litz Julien, MS, RD, LDN

Health Communications, Inc.
Deerfield Beach, Florida

www.hcibooks.com

The information contained in this book is not intended as a substitute for the advice and/or medical care of the reader's physician, nor are they meant to discourage or dissuade the reader from the advice of his or her physician. The reader should regularly consult with a physician in matters relating to his or her health and especially with regard to symptoms that may require diagnosis. Any eating or lifestyle regimen should not be undertaken without first consulting the reader's physician.

Library of Congress Cataloging-in-Publication Data
is available from the Library of Congress.

©2006 Ronni Litz Julien
ISBN 0-7573-0390-0

Publisher: Health Communications, Inc.
3201 S.W. 15th Street
Deerfield Beach, FL 33442-8190

Cover design by Larissa Hise Henoch
Inside book design by Lawna Patterson Oldfield
Cover photo ©PhotoDisc

This book is dedicated to:

- My husband and children—Stephen, Jamie and Jordan—for without their patience, their cheerleading and their computer expertise, this book would never have come to fruition.

- My parents and my in-laws—Sheila and Norman Litz and Joyce and Bruce Julien—for their constant and loving support, Sheila's editing prowess, and Joyce's years of nutritional mentoring.

- Jeannie DeQuine, my freelance editor and friend, for without your dedication, devotion and confidence, this book would have remained just a great thought.

- My agent, Bob Diforio—wouldn't be here without you.

- Chefs Michelle and Martha Bernstein for their delightful and healthful recipes.

I thank you all
from the bottom of my
trans fat free heart.
You make a difference
in my world.

Contents

Introduction

At age thirty-seven, Abby, mother of three, did not expect to be lying in the intensive care unit. She stared at the ceiling, recalling and reliving the anguish of her dad's heart attack and the many days he spent in intensive care before dying at the age of fifty-four. Abby was finally frightened.

Sure, her five-foot, five-inch frame had held about twenty-five extra pounds since her pregnancies, but otherwise, Abby felt physically well. The previous day had been a complete shock. She had entered the hospital with chest pain and, by the end of the day, had stents placed in two of her major coronary (heart) arteries.

After Abby was moved to a regular room several days later, her doctor came in to discuss the long-term changes she needed to make in her life. This is where I came in—I'm Abby's nutritionist. For several days prior to discharge, I did my best to educate her about the changes she needed to make. And they were going to be manageable ones. Of course, we discussed a low-fat diet filled with moderate amounts of healthy high fiber carbohydrates, plenty of fish, oats, olive oil and legumes. Abby was taught just how to control the larger amounts of food she wanted to eat, and for most of her life, had eaten. The most crucial change: a commitment to a regular exercise regimen—which was difficult because time was an issue—and the maintenance of a much healthier body weight. This was not negotiable.

I enlightened Abby about a newly recognized risk factor—her trans fat intake. These fats, found in so many foods—cakes, cookies, margarines and fast foods—now appear to be the most dangerous fats of all. Therefore, this was the end of Abby's "partially hydrogenated oil" or "trans fat" intake—forever.

As Abby began her new journey, she realized she was in charge of it all. And—with an awareness and some simple swaps—it can be done. Abby is living proof.

Don't Throw Out the Good with the Bad

D iseases of the heart remain the number one killer of adults in the United States, and sadly, the number of heart disease deaths seems to be increasing in our children, too. For many years, research has proven that lower fat diets, along with a few positive changes in our lifestyles, will reduce our risk of heart disease, certain cancers, diabetes and obesity. At last, we've all started to get the message.

NOT ALL FATS ARE BAD

Fat is one of six major nutrient groups, out of a long list of approximately fifty-five total nutrients, that the body needs on an ongoing basis (carbohydrate, protein and water are the other major nutrients). Fat supplies energy to the body, keeps our cells healthy, helps to regulate metabolism (the little running engine we have inside our bodies) and transports certain vitamins and minerals throughout the body. Fat also keeps our bodies insulated and warm and provides fat-soluble vitamins for proper bodily function.

Is there such a thing as consuming too little fat? Absolutely. If we do not eat enough fat, then the essential fatty acids (healthy and necessary properties of fat that help the body to function well) are limited, skin becomes flaky and itchy, and hair can begin to fall out. What is the minimal requirement? One tablespoon of oil (preferably polyunsaturated or monounsaturated) or fat per day. I bet most of us get it! Here's where some of it comes from:

- Fatty fishes
- All vegetable oils, including olive and peanut oil
- Low-fat dairy products
- Margarines

Fat is classified into two types:

- Saturated
- Unsaturated

SATURATED FATS

Saturated fats are extremely damaging fats, responsible for clogging our arteries with cholesterol, and evidently creating inflammation around our artery walls, further advancing heart disease. They are found primarily in *animal* foods: fatty and processed meats, whole milk and dairy products including ice cream and cheeses, poultry skin, and lard. Several *plant* products contain saturated fat, as well, including palm oil, palm kernel oil, coconut oil and tropical oils. These will be noted on the ingredient list of a food product (Food labels are discussed in more detail in Chapter 3). Saturated fats are solid or hard at room temperature, similar to butter in consistency. Avoid them!

UNSATURATED FATS

The second type of fat is unsaturated fat, which is soft and liquid at room temperature. In general, most unsaturated fats do not seem to be quite as destructive to our vessels. There are two groups of these:

- Polyunsaturated
- Monounsaturated

The difference between the two is their chemical makeup. When we put them into our bodies, they present different things. For years, polyunsaturated fats have been some of the safest types of fat—corn, soybean, safflower and sunflower oils. All of these contain the healthy omega-6 fats, which are found in many plant oils and nuts, specifically walnuts. And, today, it is very acceptable, even encouraged, to put nuts back on our "healthy foods" list—in small quantities, about 2 to 3 tablespoons per day. Research supports that these omega-6 fatty acids may help lower blood cholesterol levels, lower the bad LDL cholesterol, and raise the good HDL cholesterol, when substituted for saturated, or unhealthy, fat.

Omega-3: The Fishy Fat

The polyunsaturated fats talked about lately are the omega-3 fatty acids. These are primarily found in oily fish, and many studies prove that increased levels of these "omega-3s" not only lower cholesterol levels in our bloodstream, they also help to decrease inflammation in the body. Scientists suggest that it is not solely high blood cholesterol and other fats in the bloodstream that are damaging to the arteries; it is this inflammatory process as well. Recent research supports the fact that fish is the main food source that may limit this inflammation, especially in artery walls, thus helping to prevent damage.

In the year 2000, the Scientific Conference on Dietary Fatty Acids and Cardiovascular Health reported the significance of including these healthy fats in our diets regularly. Therefore, these omega-3 fatty acids, found in fish such as Pacific and Atlantic herring, Pacific mackerel, Atlantic salmon (wild), canned pink salmon, trout, oysters, whitefish, sardines and sablefish, are certainly better fat choices than the saturated versions.

My recommendation is to try to consume fish a minimum of four to five times per week. For those who are not fishlovers, flaxseed and soybean, as well as walnuts, are suggested. Fish oil supplements are recommended, especially for those who already have heart disease, a family history of heart disease, or have an aversion to fish. Because the body is incapable of making these omega-3s on its own, they must be included in our diets. The FDA suggests no more than 2 grams (2000 mg) of fish oil supplement daily. (Heed the warning about usage and dosage for pregnant and lactating women, and those on anti-clotting medications such as aspirin or Coumadin [warfarin].) For the proper dosage, please check with your medical doctor or registered/licensed dietitian. Remember to choose a reputable and regulated supplement.

So, your first order of business is to study your food labels for these ingredients and choose foods very low in saturated fats. In fact, choose foods low in total fat; therefore, you eliminate many unhealthy culprits.

Monounsaturated fats, touted as the healthiest type of fats in general, became popular several years ago, due to the benefits that were publicized by the Mediterranean diet. The high consumption of olive oil within the diets of the Greeks and Italians is considered to be one of the primary reasons why they have lower levels of heart disease. So, here in this country, we have adopted the monounsaturates: olives and olive oil, peanuts and peanut oil, rapeseed oil, avocado, and other nuts and seeds. We are highly encouraged to replace our intake of saturated fats with monounsaturated fat—certainly to help lower our cholesterol levels—and maybe even to limit our risk for certain cancers, namely breast and colon. A word of caution—all of the fats are similar in calories: about 150 per tablespoon.

With regard to cooking and food preparation, there has been a shift over the past twenty-five years from animal to vegetable fats, which, until recently, seemed to be a healthier shift. In the next chapter, we discuss which type of fat current research suggests is the worst fat of all.

What Are Trans Fats? The Worst Fat of All?

W hen a liquid oil such as corn oil is turned into a solid fat such as corn oil stick margarine, it becomes a trans fat through a process called hydrogenation—the addition of hydrogen to the liquid oil. This fat, which is now a solid, changes the basic function of our body's cells and is what researchers now feel is largely responsible for the staggering number of heart disease victims in the United States. This process of synthetically making trans fat creates a substance caustic to our systems—somewhat like ingesting plastic.

But why would manufacturers need to make a synthetic fat? After it was determined that saturated fats were so deadly, food companies chose to replace much of the saturated fats with trans fats. This is because trans fats maintain a food product's shelf life, freshness and taste. Trans fat is what makes the creamy filling in the Oreo or maintains the taste of many crackers that remain on the shelf for a long while, and it is less costly. Another reason it is added to our foods: *Fat tastes good!*

THE FACTS

Research suggests that hydrogenated products may have damaging effects similar to those of saturated fats, such as raising LDL (bad) cholesterol levels, and furthermore, lowering the HDL (good) cholesterol, causing serious injury to our heart vessels.

It is estimated that removing all trans fats from margarines and baked goods would prevent anywhere from 30,000 to 100,000 cardiac deaths a year, according to a 1999 joint report by researchers at the Harvard School of Public Health and Brigham and Women's Hospital in Boston.[1]

According to Brian Olshansky, M.D., University of Iowa Health Care professor of internal medicine, "Trans fatty acids may help preserve food so that it tastes good, but your body can't break them down and use them correctly." Dr. Olshansky claims, "Normal fats are very supple and pliable, but the trans fatty acid is a stiff fat that can build up in the body and create havoc."

In one of the early medically significant trans fat free studies published in the well-known medical journal *Lancet*, approximately 90,000 women were studied for eight years.[2] Their intake of trans fat was not incredibly high; it was just under 6 grams daily, compared with women who only ate about 2.5 grams of trans fat per day. (It doesn't take much to consume this much deadly trans fat—in May 2005 an order of french fries at a typical fast food restaurant had 8 grams of trans fat and a standard doughnut had 5 grams). Their rate of heart attack and death increased by *50 percent*, due to their trans fat intake.

Another key *Lancet* study monitored 2,033 men for two years after they suffered heart attacks and found they had a 30 percent reduction in further heart incidences by limiting trans fat and including omega-3-rich fatty fish in their diets.[3]

Several other reputable studies examining large groups of people have surfaced more recently. A study of approximately 79,000 women found they had advanced risks of coronary disease with high intakes of trans fats.[4] Most recently, studies conclude the higher intake of trans fatty acids is not just a greater cardiovascular risk, but it also increases inflammation in the body and advances the threat of diabetes, as well.

> Economically speaking, if we lower our trans fat intake, it could save an astounding $170 million to $340 million in medical costs. The country of Denmark has completely eliminated trans fat from their entire food supply and Canada and many other countries are quickly following suit.

THE STEALTH FAT

So why the fuss? Isn't it easy just to get rid of trans fats in our diets? No. Trans fats are not used solely in *unhealthy* snack items, margarines, and processed foods. Unfortunately for consumers, even those of us who think we are being "healthy" by buying products labeled "heart healthy" or "low in cholesterol" are swapping one bad choice for another, because trans fats are also found in many so-called healthier products. And even trace amounts of trans fats can add up. In addition, fast foods, french fries, salad dressings, milkshakes, hamburger and hot dog buns, breakfast foods, dry mixes for dressings, chips and breads are also on the list of foods with trans fats. So what is a consumer to do? Continue to concentrate on eating a generally low-fat diet. The target fat grams for the day in a healthy individual should be 25 to 40 total fat grams per day for adults, and 30 to 60 total fat grams for children.

In the next chapter, you will learn how to read a Nutrition Facts label, understand it, and make educated choices while shopping for you and your family. Additionally, you'll find many interesting and fun trans fat free recipes, family meal plans, information about how to make trans fat free choices when dining out, and how to keep your children trans fat free forever. You'll also find lists of brand-name, trans fat free foods to make your grocery shopping easier.

Trans Fat Free Foods and How to Find Them

We've talked about how important it is to be trans fat free. But most people don't have the time to check the labels on every item they need at the grocery store. So we've made trans fat free grocery shopping a little easier with lists of brand-name trans fat free foods. First, though, let's decode the Nutrition Facts labels.

DECIPHERING THE LABEL

Here is what to look for on the Nutrition Facts label, in trying to locate these harmful trans fats:

Nutrition Facts

Serving Size 1 cup (228g)
Servings Per Container 2

Amount per Serving

Calories 250	Calories from Fat 110

% Daily Value*

Total Fat 12g	18%
Saturated Fat 3g	15%
Trans Fat 1.5g	
Cholesterol 30mg	10%
Sodium 470mg	20%
Total Carbohydrate 31g	10%
Dietary Fiber 0g	0%
Sugar 5g	
Protein 5g	

Vitamin A	4%
Vitamin C	2%
Calcium	20%
Iron	4%

*Percent Daily Values are based on a 2,000 calorie diet. Your Daily Values may be higher or lower depending on your calorie needs:

	Calories	2,000	2,500
Total Fat	Less than	65g	80g
Sat Fat	Less than	20g	25g
Cholesterol	Less than	200mg	300g
Sodium	Less than	2,400mg	2,400mg
Total Carbohydrate		300g	275g
Dietary Fiber		25g	20g

SOME GENERAL ADVICE

In the grocery store, consider these thoughts:

• Don't judge your food just by its name. Remember that "low fat" and "cholesterol free" foods can still contain trans fat. Look for a different brand if your favorite item contains the trans fats.

• All grocery stores contain trans fat free products. You do not have to shop in a health food store.

• Try not to omit food categories because they contain trans fats. Keep looking; you will find a healthy alternative.

- Remember: Check total fat grams in a product. If it is high, you should not be choosing it often, even if it is trans fat free.
- Read the fine print on the ingredient label. You may find partially hydrogenated oils even if the product claims to be trans fat free—it is calculated on serving size.
- If you are careful with your portion sizes, you will not ingest much trans fat.

Do not allow the Nutrition Facts label to confuse you. Several numbers are important, and many others are fairly useless. In my opinion, for instance, the "Percent Daily Values" and the footnote at the bottom of the label relating to a 2,000 and 2,500 calorie diet are not universal to everyone because everyone has different needs, different activity levels and different body frame sizes, so I skip that information. Instead, pay close attention to the following label items:

- Serving Size
- Calories per serving
- Total Fat
- Saturated Fat
- Trans Fat
- Cholesterol
- Carbohydrate
- Sodium
- Fiber
- Protein

Serving Size: Many food manufacturers have learned how to dupe the consumer with this information. Learn to understand the portion size on the package, and make use of it. If you double your consumption of the recommended serving size, you must double the calories, fat, protein, and so on.

Total Fat: To set heart-healthy goals, total fat is extremely important. Healthy adult fat grams for the day are approximately **25 to 40 grams per day**; for healthy children, approximately **30 to 60 grams of fat per day**.

Saturated Fat: For many years, this was the deadliest type of fat in our diets. We should continue to be aware of our daily intakes. The latest research limits saturated fat to **10 percent of our daily calories**, or lower, if possible. What does this equate to in real life: For example, a 1,500 calorie diet (for a female adult attempting to maintain her weight, or a growing pre-teen), your saturated fat intake for the day should be no more than 150 calories (10 percent), which when divided by 9 (9 calories in 1 gram of fat) equals about 15 grams of saturated fat.

Trans Fat: The newest item to add to our list of "watch for and eliminate." The present medical and nutrition guidelines state that there is **no healthy level of trans fat acceptable in our diets**. In essence, this means to try and remove as much trans fat from your diet as possible. NOTE: *Just because a food product is trans fat free does not necessarily make it healthy. With regard to fat in general, always look for the total fat content in addition to what types of fat it contains (saturated, polyunsaturated, monounsaturated). Choose low-fat items most often.*

Cholesterol: This is found in animal products only, those that swim, walk or fly. The truth is, if we keep our total fat level on the low side, cholesterol will automatically stay low. The American Heart Association recommends no more than **300 mg of cholesterol per day** from food.

Carbohydrate: Carbohydrate is the latest nutrient under fire, so it is important to know the carb motto: Be moderate and be smart in the carbohydrate choices you make. Look for less sugar and more dietary fiber. Carbohydrates provide a well-needed source of energy to our bodies. This is not about fad diets and the radical removal of carbohydrates from our diets, and is not for diabetes prevention or weight loss, as many seem to think.

Sodium: Be aware of foods high in salt, such as canned foods, frozen meals, commercial soups, table salt, pickles, olives, processed meats and cheeses, tomato sauce and soy sauce, just to name a few. Again, the recommendations are to keep our hearts healthy by consuming no more than **2,000 to 2,400 mg sodium per day** (about 1 teaspoon of salt).

Dietary Fiber: Dietary fiber is important to keep our bowels healthy, limit the risks of colon, rectal and other cancers, improve the cholesterol levels in our bloodstream, and regulate our blood sugar levels. The goal for consumption of dietary fiber is **25 to 40 grams per day.**

Protein: This nutrient is needed for proper muscle and tissue growth and repair in our bodies, and once again, to regulate our bodies' blood sugar levels. In the United States, most of us get the adequate protein requirements: **0.5 to 1.0 gram of protein per kilogram of body weight.**

THE TRANS FAT CHEAT SHEET

- Check the ingredient labels. Read all product labels and do not buy products with the following words: "partially hydrogenated vegetable shortening," "partially hydrogenated vegetable oil" or "partially hydrogenated soybean oil."

- Purchase soft and tub margarine products that specify trans fat free, and be sure those other foods you enjoy are trans fat free as well. What makes a product trans fat free? Again, in the ingredient list, the words "partially hydrogenated vegetable oil/shortening" do *not* appear. And, avoid those stick versions of margarine at all costs.
- All ingredient lists go from what is found most in the product, down to least, in descending order. If you consume these foods occasionally, make sure that the words "partially hydrogenated oil/shortening" are at least the fifth ingredient in the label, and not the second or third.
- Choose a trans fat free margarine (such as Smart Balance— there is a version for cooking and baking), butter, or even better, a liquid oil when possible.
- The Food and Drug Administration, one of the governmental agencies overseeing our food and disease connection, has required food manufacturers to list this newly recognized "bad" fat—the trans fat grams—on the Nutrition Facts label as of January 2006.
- Watch portion sizes. Obviously, the less you consume of your favorite high fat or trans fat food, the healthier you will be.

As noted above, begin to look for the words "hydrogenated" or "partially hydrogenated vegetable oil" or "partially hydrogenated shortening" on the ingredient list, and avoid those foods. Can we completely eliminate trans fats from our lives? Probably not completely, but we can certainly try to ingest as little as possible.

THE TRULY TRANS FAT FREE TREASURES

Below you will find a list of trans fat free foods to help you get started on your quest of eliminating trans fat food from your diet. NOTE: *This extensive list of trans fat free foods compiled through September 2005.*

All beans, plain *(fresh and canned)*
All basic coffees/teas *(not necessarily the gourmet or flavored coffees)*
All eggs/all egg white products/Better 'N Eggs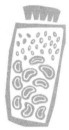
All fruits and fruit juices, fresh and canned
All Genisoy products
All Health Valley products
All jams and jellies
All meats, including beef, poultry, fish, veal, pork, lamb and organ meats
All milk products, including cottage cheese, yogurts, cheeses and sour cream
All plain/raw nuts and seeds
All pastas and noodles *(plain, not prepared)*
All fresh and frozen *(plain)* vegetables
All Whole Foods Market private labels nationwide
All Wild Oats Market private labels nationwide
All regular plain rice products

Baking Mixes, Cakes, Baking Accompaniments

Betty Crocker Low Fat Wild Blueberry Muffin Mix
Classic Hearth International Collection Bread Royal Sweet Bread
Eagle Brand Fat Free Sweetened Condensed Milk
Eagle Brand Sweetened Condensed Milk
Ghirardelli Chocolate Chip Cookie Mix

Hershey Special Dark Syrup
Hershey Strawberry Syrup
Hershey Syrup
Krusteaz Fat Free Muffin Mix
Magnolia Sweetened Condensed Milk

Beverages

Carnation Malted Milk
Choco Listo Malt Mix
Nesquik Chocolate Flavor Powdered Milk Mix
Nestle Hot Cocoa Mix, Fat Free
Ovaltine Drink Mix
Swiss Miss No Sugar Added (with Calcium) Cocoa Mix

Breads and Grain Products

Arnold's Hot Dog Buns
Arnold's Select Wheat Sandwich Rolls
Bay's English Muffins, Honey Wheat
Boboli Pizza Crust
Desde Arepas Del Paisa
La Fe Arepa Blanco
La Real Corn Tortillas
Mama Mary's Pizza Crust
Margaret's Artisan FlatBreads
Nature's Own 100% Whole Wheat Bread
Thomas' Bagels
Thomas' English Muffins
Thomas' Hearty Grain Oat Bran English Muffins
Thomas' Mini Bagels
Thomas' Mini Bagels, Cinnamon Raisin
Toufayan Onion Pita

Toufayan Pitettes
Toufayan White Pita
Toufayan Whole Wheat Pita

Candies

Brach's Jordan Almonds
Cadbury Dairy Milk Chocolate Bar
Cadbury Roast Almond Bar
Cadbury Royal Dark Chocolate Bar
Candy Corn
DOTS
Dove Milk Chocolate Miniatures
Dove Rich Dark Chocolate Miniatures
Genisoy Chocolate Soy Nuts
Hershey's Hugs
Hershey's Kisses
Hershey's Kisses with Rich Dark Chocolate
Hershey's Milk Chocolate Bar
Hershey's Nuggets
Hershey's Nuggets with Almonds
Jolly Ranchers
Jolly Ranchers Soft and Chewy Screaming Sours
Jujy Fruits
Junior Mints
Kit Kat Bars
Lindt Lindor Truffles
M&M's Peanut
M&M's Plain
Nestle Raisinets
Nestle Turtles
Pearson's Mint Patties

Reese's Peanut Butter Cups
Riesen Chocolate Caramels
Sour Patch Kids
Swedish Fish
Sweet'N Low Sugar-Free Fruit Flavored Hard Candies
Toblerone Bittersweet Chocolate Bar
Toblerone Milk Chocolate Bar
Trolli Sour Crawlers
Werther's Originals
York Peppermint Patties

Cereal and Cereal Bars

Entenmann's Multi Grain Cereal Bars
General Mills Cheerios
General Mills Cheerios Berry Burst
General Mills Cheerios Strawberry
General Mills Cheerios Triple Berry
General Mills Cheerios Vanilla
General Mills Chex (all)
General Mills Fiber One
General Mills Golden Grahams
General Mills Total Vanilla Yogurt
General Mills Wheaties
Kashi Cinnaraisin Crunch
Kashi Go Lean
Kashi Good Friends High Fiber
Kashi Heart to Heart
Kashi 7 Whole Grain Puffs
Kellogg's All Bran
Kellogg's All Bran Extra Fiber
Kellogg's Apple Jacks

Kellogg's Bran Buds
Kellogg's Complete Wheat Bran and Oat Bran
Kellogg's Corn Flakes
Kellogg's Cracklin' Oat Bran
Kellogg's Crispix
Kellogg's Frosted Flakes
Kellogg's Frosted Flakes, 1/3 Less Sugar
Kellogg's Frosted Mini Wheats
Kellogg's Kix
Kellogg's Product 19
Kellogg's Raisin Bran
Kellogg's Rice Krispies
Kellogg's Special K
Kellogg's Special K Low Carb
Kellogg's Special K Red Berries
Kellogg's Special K Vanilla Almond
Kellogg's Tiger Power
McCann's Irish Oatmeal
Nabisco Cream of Wheat Instant Original
Nabisco Cream of Wheat Maple
Post Alpha Bits
Post Bran Flakes
Post Grape Nuts
Post 100% Bran
Post Raisin Bran Cereal Bars
Post Shredded Wheat
Post Shredded Wheat 'n Bran
Quaker Instant Oatmeal
Quaker Instant Oatmeal Apple and Cinnamon
Quaker Instant Oatmeal Low Sugar Apples and Cinnamon
Quaker Instant Oatmeal Low Sugar Maple

Quaker Instant Oatmeal Maple and Brown Sugar
Quaker Instant Oatmeal Raisin Spice
Quaker Life Cereal Cinnamon
Quaker Life Cereal Whole Grain
Quaker Old Fashioned Oats
Quaker Puffed Rice
Quaker Puffed Wheat
Quaker Take Heart Golden Maple
South Beach Diet Cereal Bars
Uncle Sam
Uncle Sam Mixed Berry
Weight Watchers cereals

Condiments and Dips

All artificial sweeteners
All vinegars
Campbell's Onion Soup Mix
Dean's French Onion Dip
Dean's Lite Dips
Hellmann's Mayonnaise
Hellmann's Reduced Fat
    Mayonnaise
Kraft Mayonnaise
Kraft Miracle Whip
Lawry's Chili Seasoning
Marie's Homestyle Ranch Dip
McCormick Chicken Gravy Mix
McCormick Original Chili Seasoning
Pickles
Salsas (all)
T. Marzetti's Bacon Tomato Dip

T. Marzetti's Bleu Cheese Dip
T. Marzetti's Buffalo Ranch Dip
T. Marzetti's Dill Dip
T. Marzetti's Light Ranch Veggie Dip

Cookies

Archway Fat Free Devil's Food Cookies
Archway Fat Free Oatmeal Raisin Cookies
Back to Nature Chocolate and Mint Crème Sandwich Cookies
Back to Nature Classic Crème Sandwich Cookies
Back to Nature Crispy Oatmeal Cookies
Cascadia Farms Organic Chewy Granola Harvest Berry Bars
Health Valley Chocolate Chunk Cookies
Health Valley Mini Chocolate Chip Cookies
Health Valley Mini Chocolate Chocolate Chip Cookies
Health Valley Peanut Butter Cookies
Health Valley White Chocolate Chunk Cookies
Lance Choc-o-Lunch Cookies
Lance Van-o-Lunch Cookies
LU Le Petit Écolier Butter Biscuits with Pure Dark Chocolate
Nabisco 100 Calorie Packs Thin Crisps Oreo
Nabisco Oreos Sugar Free
Nabisco SnackWell's Cookie Cakes Black Forest
Nabisco SnackWell's Cookie Cakes Black Forest Chocolate Mint
Nabisco SnackWell's Cookie Cakes Devil's Food
Nabisco SnackWell's Devil's Food Fat Free Cookie Cakes
Nabisco Chips Ahoy! Soft Baked Chunky Chocolate Chunks
Nabisco Golden Oreos Original
Nabisco Golden Oreos Uh Oh
Newman's Own Alphabet Arrowroot Cookies
Newman's Own Alphabet Champion Chip Cookies

Newman's Own Alphabet Cinnamon Graham Cookies

Newman's Own Fig Newman's

Pepperidge Farm Soft Baked Cookies Oatmeal Cranberry

Pepperidge Farm Soft Baked Cookies Oatmeal Raisin

Pepperidge Farm Soft Baked Cookies Snickerdoodle

Pepperidge Farm Soft Baked Cookies Sugar Cookie

Pepperidge Farm Sugar Free Cookies Chocolate Chip

Pepperidge Farm Sugar Free Cookies Chocolate Chip with Pecan

Pepperidge Farm Sugar Free Cookies Milano

Voortman's Cookies

Voortman's Sugar Free Cookies

Ethnic Foods

A Taste of Thai Peanut Sauce Mix

El Sembrador Jamaican Style Patties *(frozen)*

Excelsior Fat Free Genuine Jamaican Water Crackers

Good Seasons Asian Sesame with Ginger Dressing

J. F. Mills Festival Jamaican Style Dough Mix

Joseph's Sugar Free Cookies

Kedem Tea Biscuits Chocolate Biscuits

LaUnica Toasted Bread Rolls

Manischewitz Chicken Vegetable Soup

Manischewitz Matzo Ball Mix

Manischewitz Matzo Meal

Rokeach Barley and Mushroom Soup

Santa Fe Farms Fat Free Cookies

Frozen Foods

Amy's Frozen Meals *(all)*

Bagel Bites

Bantry Bay Seafood Mussels

Boca Burgers

Catalina Ham Croquettes

Catalina Pork Tamales

Contessa Coconut Shrimp

Contessa Orange Shrimp

Contessa Thai Curry Shrimp

Cool Whip Free

Eggo 99% Fat Free Special K Waffles

Eggo Frozen Mini Pancakes

El Monterey Frozen Burritos

El Sembrador Yuca and Cheese Bread

Empire Cheese Blintzes

Empire Cherry Blintzes

Ethnic Gourmet Meals

Gardenburger Meals

Gardenburgers

Golden Blintzes

Golden Potato Pancakes

Goya All Butter Pound Cake

Goya Beef Stew with Rice Dinner

Goya Chicken Fricassee Dinner with Ham

Goya Frozen Pasteles

Goya Ground Beef, Potatoes and Seasoned Sauce with Rice Dinner

Goya Ripe Plantains

Goya Taquitos

Health is Wealth Broccoli Egg Rolls

Health is Wealth Spinach Egg Rolls

Healthy Choice Familiar Favorites Grilled White Meat
    Chicken/Mashed Potatoes

Healthy Choice Grilled Basil Chicken

Healthy Choice Grilled Whiskey Steak
Healthy Choice Lemon Pepper Fish
Healthy Choice Macaroni and Cheese
Healthy Choice Roasted Chicken Marsala
Healthy Choice Stuffed Pasta Shells
Ian's Chicken Nuggets
La Fe Corn Arepas
Lean Cuisine Balsamic Glazed Chicken
Lean Cuisine Chicken Tuscan
Lean Cuisine Lemon Garlic Shrimp
Lean Cuisine Steak Tips Dijon
Lender's Frozen Bagels
Maya Hawaiian Plantains Tostones
Meal Mart Breaded Chicken
Meal Mart Breaded Chicken Wings
Meal Mart Matzo Balls
Meal Mart Meatballs
Michael Angelo's Baked Eggplant
Michael Angelo's Chicken Alfredo
Michael Angelo's Lasagna
Michael Angelo's Vegetable Lasagna
Mon Cuisine Braised Veal
Mon Cuisine Broiled Filet of Salmon
Mon Cuisine Roast Chicken Breast
Mon Cuisine Roast Turkey
Morningstar Farms Frozen Products
Pagoda Asian Style Pork and Shrimp Egg Rolls
Pescanova Fish Fingers
Pescanova Squid Rings
Pescanova Whiting Croquettes
Quorn Meat Free Dinners

Ratner's Blintzes
Ratner's Potato Pirogen
Rubashkin's Aaron's Best Beef Patties
Sea Pak Jumbo Butterfly Shrimp
Sea Pak Popcorn Shrimp
Stouffer's Salisbury Steak
Tabatchnik Frozen Soups

Ice Cream and Frozen Desserts

Ben & Jerry's Body and Soul Ice Creams (*all flavors*)
Ben & Jerry's Chocolate Chip Cookie Dough Ice Cream
Ben & Jerry's Oatmeal Cookie Ice Cream
Breyer's Carb Smart Ice Cream
Breyer's Heart Smart Ice Cream
Edy's No Sugar Added Fat Free Ice Cream
Edy's No Sugar Added Ice Cream
Edy's Whole Fruit Fruit Bars
Eskimo Pie Pops
Fudgsicles
Häagen-Dazs (*all flavors*)
Häagen-Dazs Lite (*all flavors*)
Healthy Choice Premium Low Fat Vanilla Ice Cream
Klondike Slim-a-Bear
Nabisco Chocolate Flavor Ice Cream Cones
Nestle Double Fudge Pop
Philly Swirl Fruit Juice Swirls
Popsicle Brand Popsicles
Snickers Ice Cream Bars
Starbucks Frappucino Café Vanilla Bars
Starbucks Frappucino Low Fat Mocha Bars
Tropicana Orange Cream Bars

Whole Fruit Sorbet and Bars

Infant Formulas and Baby Food

Beech-Nut Baby Foods and Cereals

Beech-Nut Table Time Baby Foods

Enfamil Formulas

Gerber Baby Foods and Cereals

Gerber Finger Foods Fruit Wagon Wheels

Gerber Graduates Banana Cereal Snackin' Squares

Gerber Graduates Li'l Entrees

Gerber Graduates Mini Veggies Bite Size Freeze Dried Snacks

Gerber Tender Harvest Baby Foods

Nestle Good Start Formulas

Pediasure

Similac Formulas

Miscellaneous

Rothbury Farms Seasoned Croutons

Oils, Margarines, Spreads

Earth Balance Natural Buttery Spread

Promise Butter Spread

Smart Balance Buttery Spread

Smart Balance Buttery Spread Light

Smart Squeeze Margarine Spread

Pasta Products

All Buitoni products

All DaVinci products

All DiGiorno products

Gia Russa Noodle Products
Gia Russa Tortellini Egg Pasta (*cheese*)
Gia Russa Tortellini Egg Pasta (*spinach*)
Kraft Macaroni and Cheese
Monterey Pasta Company Whole Wheat Ravioli/Tortellini

Peanut Butter

Skippy Natural Peanut Butter
Smart Balance Omega Natural Peanut Butter
Smucker's Natural Chunky Peanut Butter
Smucker's Natural Creamy Peanut Butter

Popcorn

Newman's Own Natural Popcorn
Smart Balance Light Butter Popcorn
Smart Balance Movie Style Popcorn

Prepared Foods, Canned Foods

Bush's Baked Beans
Fantastic Vegetarian Sloppy Joe Mix
Lipton Cajun Sides
Lipton Fiesta Sides Taco Rice
Lipton Rice Sides
Mama Mary's Pancakes

Refrigerated Products

Goya Prepared Corn Pudding
Goya Prepared Flan
Jell-O Fat Free Sugar Free Puddings
Kozy Shack Puddings

Vita Herring in Sour Cream Sauce
Vita Herring Tidbits in Wine Sauce

Salad Dressings, Marinades, Seasoning Mixes

Cardini's Balsamic Vinaigrette Dressing
Cardini's Caesar Dressing
Cardini's Fat Free Dressings
Cardini's Poppy Seed Dressing
Heinz Salad Cream
Hidden Valley Caesar Dressing
Hidden Valley Fat Free Dressings
Hidden Valley French Dressing
Hidden Valley Lite Ranch Dressing
Hidden Valley Ranch Dressing
House-Autry Original Recipe Seafood Breader
Kellogg's Corn Flake Crumbs
Ken's Dressings
Ken's Fat Free Dressings
Ken's Lite Dressings
Kentucky Kernel Seasoned Flour
Kraft Free Dressings
Kraft Seven Seas Italian Dressing
Kraft Special Collection Balsamic Vinaigrette Dressing
Kraft Thousand Island Dressing
Maple Grove Farms of Vermont Fat Free Dressings
Maple Grove Farms of Vermont Lite Dressings
Nabisco Cracker Meal
Newman's Own Dressings
Old Bay Seafood Seasoning
Original Trenton Cracker OTC Cracker Meal
Quaker Yellow Corn Meal

Silver Palate Creamy Caesar Salad Dressing
Silver Palate Great Goddess
Silver Palate Organic Red Wine with Olive Oil Dressing
Silver Palate Salad Splashes
Wish-Bone Deluxe Good Honey Dijon Low Fat Dressing
Wish-Bone Fat Free Dressings
Wish-Bone House Italian Dressing
Wish-Bone Just 2 Good Bleu Cheese Dressing
Wish-Bone Ranch Dressing
Wondra Flour and Gravy Mix

Snacks and Crackers

All marshmallows
Annie's Cheddar Bunnies
Back to Nature Classic Rounds
Back to Nature Crispy Wheats
Back to Nature White Cheddar Rice Thins
Baked Lays Potato Chips
Baked Ruffles Potato Chips
Betty Crocker Fruit Smoothie Fruit Snacks
Cape Cod Potato Chips
Cape Cod Reduced Fat Potato Chips
Carr's Rosemary Crackers
Carr's Whole Wheat Crackers
David Pumpkin Seeds
David Sunflower Seeds Original
"Dirty" Potato Chips
Entenmann's Little Bites (all)
Fritos Scoops
Gilda Mini Toast
Hunt's Snack Pack Fat Free Pudding

Kashi TLC Country Cheddar Crackers

Kashi TLC Honey Sesame Crackers

Kashi TLC Ranch Crackers

Kashi TLC Seven Grain Crackers

Kashi Trail Mix Chewy Granola Bars

Kashi Trail Mix Honey Almond Flax Bars

Kavli Crispy Thin Crackers

Kavli Hearty Thick Crackers

Kellogg's Nutri Grain Cereal Bars Apple Cinnamon

Kellogg's Nutri Grain Cereal Bars Mixed Berry

Kellogg's Nutri Grain Cereal Bars Raspberry

Kraft Cheese Nips Baked Snacks Cheddar Reduced Fat

Kraft Cheese Nips Baked Snacks Fairly Odd Parents

Kraft Cheese Nips Baked Snacks Four Cheese

Kraft Cheese Nips Oven Toasted Bold Cheddar

Kraft Cheese Nips Oven Toasted Nacho

Kraft South Beach Diet Snack Crackers

Nabisco Capri Sun Sour Juicers Fruit Snacks

Nabisco Kid Sense Fun Packs Cheese Nips

Nabisco Kid Sense Fun Packs Cubs Cinnamon

Nabisco Kid Sense Fun Packs Ritz Bits

Nabisco Kid Sense Fun Packs Sports Crisps

Nabisco Kid Sense Fun Packs Teddy Grahams

Nabisco Triscuits Deli Style Rye

Nabisco Triscuits Low Sodium

Nabisco Triscuits Multi Grain

Nabisco Triscuits Original

Nabisco Triscuits Reduced Fat

Nabisco Triscuits Thin Crisps

Nabisco Wheat Thins Original

Nabisco Wheat Thins Ranch

Nabisco Wheat Thins Reduced Fat
Nature Valley Chewy Trail Mix Variety Pack
Nature Valley Crunchy Granola Bars Variety Pack
New York Flatbreads Fat Free Crackers
New York Flatbreads Garlic Crackers
Old London Melba Toast White
Old London Melba Toast Whole Grain
Pepperidge Farm Goldfish Baked Snack Crackers
Pepperidge Farm Snack Sticks
Pringles BBQ Flavor Crisps
Pringles Fat Free Potato Crisps
Pringles Potato Crisps
Pringles Reduced Fat Original Crisps
Quaker Crunch Granola Snack Bars
Quaker Rice Cakes Apple Cinnamon Cakes
Quaker Rice Cakes Caramel Corn Cakes
Quaker Quakes Chocolate Rice Cakes
Quaker Soy Crisps
Ritz Chips Oven Toasted Cheddar
Ritz Chips Oven Toasted Sour Cream
Robert's American Gourmet Smart Puffs
Royal Sire Sourdough Thin Pretzels
Ruffles Light Potato Chips
RyKrisp Crackers
Seneca Crispy Apple Chips Caramel
Seneca Crispy Apple Chips Cinnamon
Seneca Crispy Apple Chips Granny Smith
Seneca Crispy Apple Chips Original
Seneca Crispy Apple Chips Sour Apple
Seneca Crispy Sweet Potato Chips Cinnamon
Seneca Crispy Sweet Potato Chips Sea Salt

Snapea Crisps
Snyder's Pretzels
Stretch Island 100% Fruit Leather
Sun Chips
Sunkist Almond Accents Butter Toffee
Sunkist Almond Accents Italian Parmesan
Sunkist Almond Accents Original
Sunkist Almond Munchies Buttered Up
Sunkist Almond Munchies Honey Dipped
Sunkist Almond Munchies Roasty Toasty
Sunkist Nuts
Terra Chips
The Snack Factory Pretzel Chips (all)
Tostitos Bite Size White Corn Chips
Wasa Crackers
Wise BBQ Chips
Wise Ridgies Potato Chips

Soups

Campbell's Bean and Bacon Soup
Campbell's Chicken with Rice Soup
Campbell's French Onion Soup
Campbell's Green Pea Soup
Campbell's Just Heat and Sip Chicken and Stars
Campbell's Just Heat and Sip Chicken with Mini Noodles
Campbell's Minestrone Soup
Campbell's Onion Soup Mix
Campbell's Oyster Stew Soup
Campbell's Tomato Noodle Soup
Health Valley Soups
Healthy Choice Chicken Noodle Soup

Healthy Choice Chicken with Rice Soup
Healthy Choice Country Vegetable Soup
Nissin Cup Noodles
Progresso Traditional 99% Fat Free Soups
Progresso Traditional Chicken Rice Soup
Progresso Traditional Southwestern Style Corn Chowder
Progresso Vegetable Classics Cheese and Herb Tortellini Soup

Soy and Tofu Products

Edamame
Lightlife veggie protein products
Nasoya Tofu products
Yves Veggie Cuisine

Sports and Nutrition Bars

AdvantEdge Bars
Balance Bars
Balance Carb Well Bars
Balance Gold Bars
Clif Bars
Genisoy Soy Protein Bars
Hershey's Smart Zone Bars
Luna Bars
Power Bar
Power Bar Harvest
Power Bar Protein Plus Carb Select
Pria Bars
Pria Carb Select
Protein Plus Carb Select
Zone Perfect Bars

Tomato Sauces

Barilla Basilico Sauce
Barilla Campagnola Roasted Garlic and Onion Sauce
Bertolli Pasta Sauces
Emeril's Pasta Sauces
Prego Hearty Meat Sauces
Prego 100% Natural Pasta Sauces
Prego 100% Traditional Pasta Sauces
Prego Organic Pasta Sauces
Ragu Old World Style Sauces
Ragu Old World Style Sauce Flavored with Meat

Yogurts

All Dannon products
All Hood Carb Countdown products
All La Yogurt products
All Yoplait products

Cooking
Trans Fat Free

Enjoy the delicious and easy trans fat free recipes on the following pages. You can rest comfortably knowing you and your family are preserving your hearts for healthier and longer lives.

When using your favorite family recipes that might contain trans fats, consider these trans fat free substitutes:

- Smart Balance
- Enova Oil
- Canola or olive oil
- Earth Balance
- Promise

Appetizers

Tomatoes Rockefeller

Serves 4

2 large vine-ripe tomatoes
½ cup Kellogg's corn flake
crumbs

½ cup Seabrook Farms creamed
spinach
2 tsps Worcestershire sauce

Preheat oven to 350 degrees. Slice tomatoes in half, and slice off a small piece from the bottom of the tomato so it sits well. Mix together corn flake crumbs, spinach and Worcestershire sauce. Place on top of tomatoes. Bake for 10 to15 minutes or until crisp.

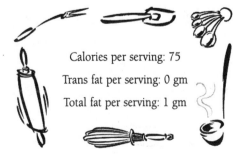

Calories per serving: 75

Trans fat per serving: 0 gm

Total fat per serving: 1 gm

Black Bean Dip

Serves 15

2 cans Progresso black beans,
  drained
2 cans Green Giant Mexicorn,
  drained
4 scallions, minced
¼ cup olive oil

½ cup vinegar
1 tomato, diced
1 avocado, diced
1 (10 oz.) bag Baked Tostitos
Dollop of Dannon plain
  low-fat yogurt

Mix beans, corn and scallions. Blend oil and vinegar, add to bean-corn mixture and refrigerate for 3 hours. Then, add diced avocado and tomato to mixture, stirring gently. Serve with trans fat free Baked Tostitos.

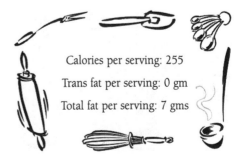

Calories per serving: 255
Trans fat per serving: 0 gm
Total fat per serving: 7 gms

Artichoke Dip

Serves 10 to 12

1 (10 oz.) can artichoke hearts in water, drained

1 cup Hellmann's low-fat mayonnaise or canola oil mayonnaise

1 cup low-fat shredded mozzarella cheese

1 cup Kraft Parmesan cheese

1/2 tsp garlic powder

Dash paprika

Preheat oven to 350 degrees. Combine artichokes, mayonnaise, mozzarella cheese, Parmesan cheese and garlic powder. Spread mixture in a small casserole dish. Sprinkle with paprika. Bake for 30 minutes or until bubbly and lightly browned. Serve with Carr's or Nabisco crackers.

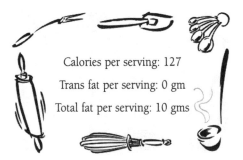

Calories per serving: 127

Trans fat per serving: 0 gm

Total fat per serving: 10 gms

Spinach and Goat Cheese Pizza

Serves 8

1 (12 inch) Boboli pizza crust	3½ ounces goat cheese
1 Tbsp olive oil	PAM cooking spray
1 cup shredded low-fat	1 Tbsp mustard seed
mozzarella cheese	18 fresh small spinach leaves

Preheat oven to 500 degrees. Brush pizza crust with olive oil. Cover with mozzarella cheese and sprinkle with goat cheese. In small skillet, spray cooking spray and sauté mustard seed until it pops. Sprinkle over the pizza. Arrange the spinach leaves. Bake in oven 10 to 12 minutes.

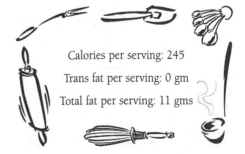

Calories per serving: 245

Trans fat per serving: 0 gm

Total fat per serving: 11 gms

Sliced Baked Salami

Serves 10 to 12

2 pound Hebrew National
Lean Salami

1 cup barbeque sauce
1 cup Chinese sweet and sour sauce

Preheat oven to 325 degrees. Make small slits on the top of the salami with a knife. Spread sauces on top. Bake for about 45 to 60 minutes, basting throughout.

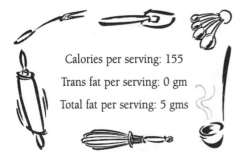

Calories per serving: 155

Trans fat per serving: 0 gm

Total fat per serving: 5 gms

Hot Crab Dip

Serves 10 to 12

16 ounces low-fat cream cheese
8 ounces low-fat sour cream
4 Tbsp Hellmann's reduced fat
   mayonnaise
1 tsp dry mustard

½ tsp lemon juice
⅛ tsp garlic salt
1 pound fresh crabmeat
1 cup 2% reduced fat shredded
   cheddar cheese

Preheat oven to 325 degrees. Blend all ingredients (except crabmeat and half the cheese) in a blender/food processor. Fold in crabmeat. Place in casserole dish. Bake for 45 minutes. Add remainder of cheese on top and sprinkle paprika. Continue baking for 10 minutes. Serve with whole grain crackers.

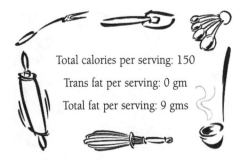

Total calories per serving: 150

Trans fat per serving: 0 gm

Total fat per serving: 9 gms

Crispy Garlic Pita Chips and Hummus

Serves 16

4 Tbsp olive oil	Salt to taste
1 clove garlic, crushed	PAM cooking spray
1 package Toufayan pita bread	2 pounds hummus

Preheat oven to 350 degrees. Combine olive oil and garlic. Cut each pita into six pieces. Brush pita pieces with olive oil. Lightly sprinkle with salt. Spray baking sheet with PAM. Place in single layer onto baking sheet and bake for approximately 20 minutes. Serve warm or at room temperature with hummus.

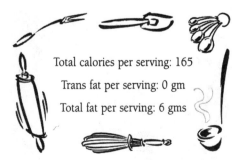

Total calories per serving: 165

Trans fat per serving: 0 gm

Total fat per serving: 6 gms

Chopped Eggplant

Serves 16

4 whole eggplant	3 Tbsp Hellmann's reduced-fat
6 hard-boiled eggs	mayonnaise
2 Tbsp onion, finely grated	Salt to taste

Peel eggplant and cut into large chunks. Place into a pot with small amount of water. Boil eggplant until very soft. Drain in strainer until all liquid is removed. Mash hard-boiled eggs; add grated onion, mayonnaise and salt to taste. Mash eggplant until almost puréed. Add to egg mixture. Mix well and refrigerate. Remove any liquid before serving. Garnish with radishes. Serve with Pepperidge Farm Snack Sticks or Nabisco Wheat Thins.

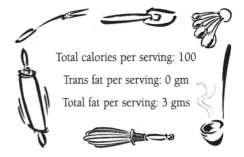

Total calories per serving: 100

Trans fat per serving: 0 gm

Total fat per serving: 3 gms

Entrées

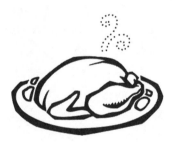

Grilled Chicken Citrus

Serves 4

5 medium oranges
½ cup barbeque sauce

4 small boneless skinless chicken
breast halves

Squeeze juice from 3 oranges, mix with the barbeque sauce. Pour half of the mixture into large resealable plastic bag. Add the chicken, seal the bag and marinate (place on the bottom shelf of your refrigerator) for at least one hour. Refrigerate the additional sauce.

Remove the chicken from the marinade, and discard the marinade. Heat grill. Place the 3 remaining oranges, peeled and sliced, on the grill along with the chicken. Cook chicken through, brushing remaining sauce onto the chicken. Place chicken on a serving dish, layering the grilled oranges on top.

NOTE: *Serve with a Caesar salad garnished with grape tomatoes, Ken's Lite Caesar dressing, and corn on the cob for a colorful, high fiber, tasty barbeque.*

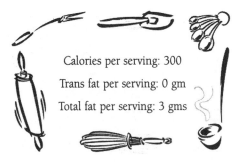

Calories per serving: 300

Trans fat per serving: 0 gm

Total fat per serving: 3 gms

Chicken Curry

Serves 6

Chef Michelle Bernstein
Miami, Florida

2 (8 oz.) containers
  low-fat plain yogurt
2 Tbsp curry powder
3 cloves crushed garlic

1 tsp chopped basil
1 tsp chopped mint
Salt to taste
6 skinless chicken breasts

Mix yogurt, curry powder, garlic, basil and mint in a bowl, stirring with a wooden spoon. Submerge chicken breasts into the sauce, cover, and refrigerate for 3 to 24 hours. Spray grill with olive oil, and cook chicken for 5 to 7 minutes on each side.

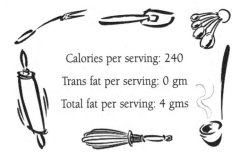

Calories per serving: 240

Trans fat per serving: 0 gm

Total fat per serving: 4 gms

Poached Chicken with
Sweet Calabaza and Sizzling Oil

Serves 4

Chef Michelle Bernstein
Miami, Florida

FOR THE CHICKEN:

64 oz. defatted chicken stock
1 Tbsp peeled and chopped
   ginger
1 whole star anise

1 Tbsp chopped lemongrass
1 Tbsp chopped garlic
2 pounds chicken, skinned,
   cut in quarters

FOR THE CALABAZA (PUMPKIN SQUASH):

1 Tbsp grapeseed oil
1 Tbsp brown sugar
pinch of cinnamon
1 tsp vanilla extract

¼ calabaza, or pumpkin squash,
   peeled and cut into 1-inch
   cubes
Salt and black pepper to taste

FOR THE SIZZLING OIL:

1 tsp peanut oil
1 Tbsp thinly sliced scallions
1 Tbsp peeled and julienne ginger

1 tsp soy sauce
1 tsp sherry vinegar

Preheat oven to 350 degrees. Combine the chicken stock, ginger, star anise, garlic and lemongrass. Bring to a boil, reduce to a simmer, and add the chicken. Cook 20 to 30 minutes.

(*continued on next page*)

Prepare the calabaza. Blend the oil, brown sugar, cinnamon and vanilla together with a whisk. Coat the calabaza with the mixture, place it on a cookie sheet and cover it with foil. Bake the calabaza until tender and golden, 35 to 45 minutes, removing the foil for the last 10 minutes. Season with salt and pepper.

To make the sizzling oil, heat the peanut oil in a sauté pan until oil just smokes. Remove from the heat and quickly add the scallions and ginger. After 30 seconds, add the soy sauce and vinegar, shaking the pan so that nothing burns. To serve, place the chicken on top of the calabaza and quickly pour the sizzling oil over the chicken. Serve immediately.

NOTE: *Serve with a large colorful field green salad with red onions, and a serving of brown rice for a diverse blend of flavors, colors, and nutrients.*

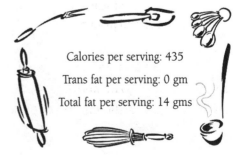

Calories per serving: 435

Trans fat per serving: 0 gm

Total fat per serving: 14 gms

Chicken Fingers with Honey Mustard

Serves 6

HONEY MUSTARD SAUCE:

½ cup honey

¼ cup Dijon mustard

CHICKEN FINGERS:

4 chicken breasts, skinless
    and boneless
1 cup all-purpose flour
½ tsp salt

¼ tsp pepper
¾ cup low-fat milk
    (or 3 to 4 egg whites)
¼ cup olive oil

Prepare the honey mustard sauce one or two days ahead for a more pungent flavor. Keep in refrigerator.

Cut chicken into strips. Mix flour, salt and pepper in a shallow bowl. Dip chicken in milk (or egg whites). Roll in flour mixture and coat well. Place chicken on waxed paper. Place oil in bottom of frying pan and fry chicken strips until golden brown. Serve with sauce.

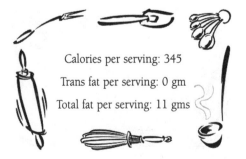

Calories per serving: 345

Trans fat per serving: 0 gm

Total fat per serving: 11 gms

NOTE: *Serve with chopped cucumber and tomato salad, baked sweet potato wedges and fresh sautéed broccoli for cancer-preventing fiber, antioxidants and phyto-chemicals.*

Spicy Chicken

Serves 6

2 pounds chicken, skinless,
   boneless and chopped
1 to 2 Tbsp peanut oil
2 Tbsp chopped scallions
1 clove garlic
2 Tbsp minced fresh ginger
1 cup sliced red pepper
3 Tbsp dry sherry

½ cup chili sauce
¼ cup ketchup
2 to 3 Tbp light soy sauce
½ tsp to 1 Tbsp hot pepper sauce
   (add slowly to taste)
1 tsp sugar
1 cup peanuts or walnuts

Sauté chicken in peanut oil until cooked through and slightly browned. Transfer to a plate. Add scallions, garlic, ginger and pepper to the oil; cook until soft. Add the other ingredients except the chicken and peanuts. Stir well and remove from the heat. Add chicken and peanuts. Serve immediately.

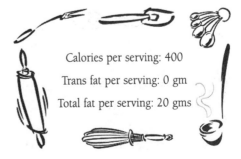

Calories per serving: 400
Trans fat per serving: 0 gm
Total fat per serving: 20 gms

Honey Apple Glazed Turkey Breast

Serves 10

1 Tbsp canola oil
⅓ cup honey
1 Tbsp dry mustard
1 (6 oz.) can frozen apple juice
  concentrate

2 tsp salt
1 tsp pepper
1 clove garlic
4 to 5 pound turkey breast

Preheat oven to 325 degrees. For the glaze, combine oil, honey, mustard and apple juice concentrate in a small bowl. Stir well and set aside. Sprinkle turkey with seasonings and garlic, and rub into the turkey. Place turkey on a rack in a roasting pan. Cover with foil and bake for 1 hour. Uncover, add the glaze and bake for an additional 1 hour. Let cool for 10 minutes.

NOTE: *Serve with spinach salad with strawberries and sliced almonds, and a mashed sweet potato, offering a delicious meal filled with potassium, vitamin C, iron, and cancer and heart-disease fighting nutrients.*

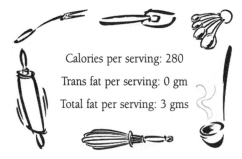

Calories per serving: 280

Trans fat per serving: 0 gm

Total fat per serving: 3 gms

Mediterranean Style Turkey "Meat" Balls and Sauce

Serves 6 to 8

Chef Michelle Bernstein
Miami, Florida

MEATBALL INGREDIENTS:

2 pounds lean ground turkey breast	3 cloves garlic
	2 Tbsp fresh parsley
1 egg	2 Tbsp fresh basil
2 Tbsp Parmesan cheese	2 Tbsp mint
2 slices of Nature's Own 100%	1/2 tsp salt
whole wheat bread *(cut off crust)*,	1 tsp paprika
soak in 2 oz. low-fat milk	Juice of 1/2 lemon

Preheat oven to 350 degrees. Chop above ingredients (with exception of the turkey breast) in a food processor. Add the turkey breast and mix well. Roll into small balls and place on a cookie sheet, sprayed with cooking spray.

(continued on next page)

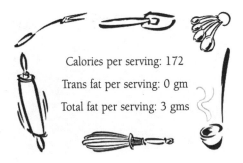

Calories per serving: 172

Trans fat per serving: 0 gm

Total fat per serving: 3 gms

SAUCE INGREDIENTS:

1 jar Bertolli or Prego spaghetti   3 Tbsp Parmesan cheese
   sauce
½ cup white wine *(optional)*

Heat sauce until very hot. Add wine and lower the heat. Drop the meatballs into the sauce. Sprinkle Parmesan cheese on top. Simmer for 30 minutes and serve.

NOTE: *Serve with tossed green salad with butter lettuce, and whole wheat pasta for a high-carotenoid (antioxidants from tomato sauce) and a high-fiber meal.*

Sautéed Snapper with Kiwi

Serves 4

Chef Michelle Bernstein
Miami, Florida

3 Tbsp olive oil
4-7 ounce fillets of snapper
2 shallots, julienne
4 kiwis, peeled and sliced into
   5 pieces each

1 Tbsp chopped mint
1 lemon, cut in half
1 Tbsp butter

In large frying pan, heat olive oil. When hot, place the snapper in the pan. Cook about 4 minutes on each side. When about three-quarters done, add the shallots and cook for about 1 minute. Add the kiwis, mint, and lemon juice from the lemon, and drizzle the butter. Shake the pan so that the sauce coats the fish. Serve immediately.

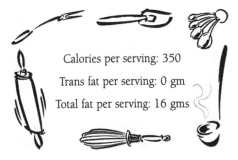

Calories per serving: 350
Trans fat per serving: 0 gm
Total fat per serving: 16 gms

Asian Salmon

Serves 4

2 Tbsp olive or canola oil	1 Tbsp ginger
2 Tbsp light soy sauce	½ tsp dry mustard
2 Tbsp lemon juice	1½ pounds salmon fillet
1 Tbsp garlic powder	

Mix marinade ingredients *(all except fish)*. Pour over fish and refrigerate for 2 hours. Preheat oven to 400 degrees. Place fish on baking sheet and bake for 30 minutes.

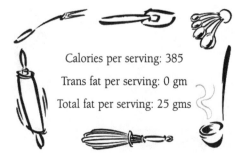

Calories per serving: 385

Trans fat per serving: 0 gm

Total fat per serving: 25 gms

Easy Baked Fish

Serves 4

4 Tbsp canola oil
½ cup dry white wine
4 Tbsp fresh squeezed lemon juice
1 to 2 large ripe tomatoes,
   thinly sliced
½ cup Kellogg's corn flake crumbs

1½ pounds thin whitefish fillet
   (sole, grouper, snapper, trout)
Salt and pepper to taste
1 clove garlic
Sprinkle of paprika

Preheat oven to 400 degrees. In small saucepan, bring oil, wine and lemon juice to a boil. Remove from heat to cool. In shallow baking dish, place a layer each of sliced tomato and corn flake crumbs, then place fish on top. Pour oil and wine mixture on the fish. Sprinkle with salt and pepper, and add garlic. Sprinkle with paprika. Bake for 15 to 20 minutes.

NOTE: *Serve with lightly sautéed broccoli and baked potato wedges for lots of fiber and omega-3 fats (from the fish).*

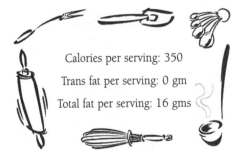

Calories per serving: 350
Trans fat per serving: 0 gm
Total fat per serving: 16 gms

Shrimply Delicious

Serves 4

¼ cup all-purpose flour
1 clove garlic, minced
½ tsp salt
⅛ tsp pepper
1 pound raw shrimp, peeled and
  deveined
4 Tbsp olive or canola oil

1 (16 oz.) can stewed tomatoes
½ cup chopped green chili peppers
  (optional)
¼ cup dry sherry
1½ cups cooked brown rice
Parsley, to garnish

Combine flour, garlic, salt and pepper. Roll shrimp in flour mixture. Heat oil on low heat. Fry shrimp until lightly browned. Add tomatoes, chili peppers and sherry; heat thoroughly, stirring occasionally. Serve over brown rice. Garnish with parsley.

NOTE: *Add mixed leafy green salad and steamed green beans for a beautifully colored, high fiber, omega-3-rich meal.*

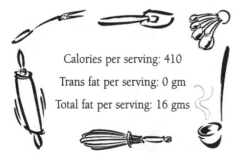

Calories per serving: 410
Trans fat per serving: 0 gm
Total fat per serving: 16 gms

Grilled Tuna Steaks
with Onion Dill "Butter" Sauce

Serves 4

¼ cup Promise margarine	2 pounds small new red potatoes,
¼ cup finely chopped onion	quartered
1 tbsp dried dill weed	2 pounds tuna steaks

Prepare a hot grill. In a small bowl, prepare onion dill butter sauce by melting margarine and adding onion and dill. Place potatoes in the center of an 18-inch square *(approximately)* piece of heavy-duty aluminum foil. Drizzle with small amount of butter mixture. Bring edges of foil together, and tightly seal top and sides. Place the potato bundle on the grill 20 to 30 minutes, or until tender.

Brush tuna steaks with remaining butter mixture. Place fish on grill during last 15 minutes of grilling time, until fish flakes with a fork.

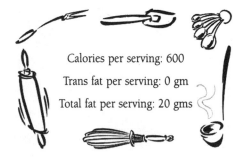

Calories per serving: 600
Trans fat per serving: 0 gm
Total fat per serving: 20 gms

Veal Marsala

Serves 4

4 Tbsp flour	4 medium shallots, chopped
salt and pepper to taste	1 pound veal cutlets
1 tsp garlic powder	²/₃ cup Marsala wine
2 tsp olive oil	½ cup water

Mix flour and salt and pepper. Heat oil in a nonstick skillet on medium-high. Sauté shallots about 2 minutes. Coat both sides of the veal with flour, shaking off the excess; add to the skillet. Sauté veal one minute per side and remove; it should be almost cooked through.

Raise heat to high, add the Marsala wine and ¼ cup water to the skillet. Bring to a boil for 1 minute. Remove pan from the heat. Place the veal in the wine sauce, turning so it is completely coated with sauce. Pour sauce on the veal when serving.

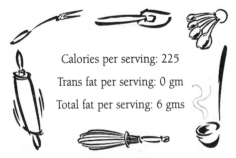

Calories per serving: 225

Trans fat per serving: 0 gm

Total fat per serving: 6 gms

Glazed Pork Medallions

Serves 4

1 ½ pounds pork tenderloin	4 tsp Dijon mustard
4 Tbsp maple syrup	2 tsp olive oil
4 Tbsp balsamic vinegar	

Remove fat from the pork and cut into 1-inch slices. Place slices between 2 pieces of plastic wrap and flatten to ½-inch thickness. Whisk the maple syrup, balsamic vinegar and mustard together. Heat olive oil in a nonstick skillet on high. Brown the pork medallions for 2 minutes. Turn and brown other side for another 2 minutes. Reduce heat to low, pour maple syrup mixture over pork, cover with a lid, and cook 2 minutes. Spoon sauce on top.

NOTE: *Serve with lightly sautéed broccoli or spinach and corn on the cob for a colorful, high fiber cancer fighting meal!*

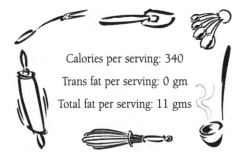

Calories per serving: 340

Trans fat per serving: 0 gm

Total fat per serving: 11 gms

Fabulous Grilled Flank Steak

Serves 4

1½ pound flank steak
3 Tbsp ketchup

3 Tbsp brown sugar
clove of garlic

Marinate steak in ketchup, brown sugar and garlic for 2 hours. Place on grill 3 to 4 minutes each side.

NOTE: *Serve with Caesar salad, low-fat Cardini's dressing, sprinkled Parmesan cheese, and a baked potato with the skin, for a potassium-rich, high-iron, vitamin B_{12}-rich delicious meal.*

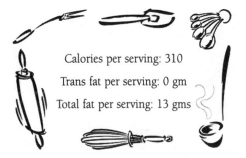

Calories per serving: 310

Trans fat per serving: 0 gm

Total fat per serving: 13 gms

Lean Mean Chili

Serves 10 to 12

PAM cooking spray
2 medium onions, chopped
2 cloves garlic, crushed
1 green pepper, chopped
3 pounds lean ground sirloin
1 package Lawry's chili
  seasoning mix

1 jar tomato sauce
1 small can tomato purée
½ cup ketchup
1 large can kidney beans
1 can beer *(optional)*
Salt and pepper to taste

Sauté onion, garlic and green pepper in cooking spray until transparent. Brown the beef until thoroughly cooked. Continue to stir. Add seasoning mix, tomato sauce, tomato purée and ketchup. Stir well. Add beer and kidney beans. Simmer for 20 minutes.

NOTE: *Serve with sliced tomato and onion salad and brown rice for a high-fiber, high-beta-carotene, spicy and flavorful meal.*

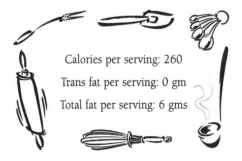

Calories per serving: 260

Trans fat per serving: 0 gm

Total fat per serving: 6 gms

Meat Loaf

Serves 6 to 8

1 small can tomato sauce	⅓ cup brown sugar
1 small onion	1 egg
¼ cup Kellogg's corn flake crumbs	Salt and pepper to taste
	1 Tbsp parsley
Juice of 1 lemon	2 pounds lean ground beef

Preheat oven to 350 degrees. In a food processor, combine all ingredients except meat. Add meat by kneading with your hands. Mix well. Shape into a loaf, glaze with a small amount of ketchup, and bake for 1 hour.

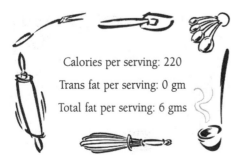

Calories per serving: 220

Trans fat per serving: 0 gm

Total fat per serving: 6 gms

Luscious Lasagna

Serves 8 to 10

1 pound ground sirloin
1 pound ground veal
PAM cooking spray
1 large onion, chopped
²/₃ cup green pepper, chopped
½ pound fresh sliced mushrooms
1 tsp salt
½ tsp pepper
1 tsp oregano

2 cans (10 oz.) Campbell's
   condensed tomato soup
1 can (6 oz.) tomato paste
²/₃ cup water
2 Tbsp Worcestershire sauce
8 ounces lasagna noodles
½ pound reduced fat shredded
   cheddar cheese

Preheat oven to 375 degrees. Spray nonstick cooking spray in a skillet. Brown meat, then add onion, green pepper, mushrooms and salt and pepper. Cook until tender, about 5 minutes. In a blender, mix oregano, tomato soup, tomato paste, water and Worcestershire sauce. Cook noodles in boiling water until almost tender. Drain and rinse. In a large, greased baking dish, spread half the noodles, cover with half of meat and sauce mixture, and sprinkle with half the cheese, repeat process, using remaining ingredients. Bake for 45 minutes or until hot.

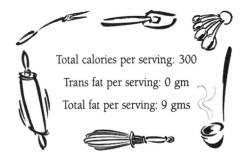

Total calories per serving: 300

Trans fat per serving: 0 gm

Total fat per serving: 9 gms

Vegetables

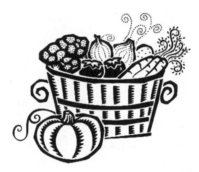

Tropical Green Beans

Serves 6 to 8

2 Tbsp olive oil	3 stalks hearts of palm, cut into
1 pound fresh green beans,	½ inch rings
cleaned and cut	⅓ cup diced sun-dried tomatoes
1 small yellow onion, cut in rings	2 tsp toasted pine nuts
6 garlic cloves, peeled and halved	Freshly ground black pepper
½ tsp salt	to taste
2 Tbsp balsamic vinegar	

Preheat oven to 400 degrees. Brush a large baking dish with 1 tablespoon of the olive oil. Put green beans, onion and garlic in dish; drizzle with remaining tablespoon of olive oil and sprinkle with salt. Bake for 25 minutes, stirring the green beans. Remove beans from oven and transfer to a serving dish. Immediately drizzle with vinegar. Add hearts of palm, tomatoes, pine nuts and pepper to taste. Toss and serve.

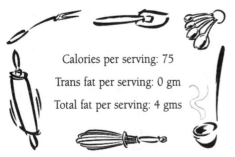

Calories per serving: 75

Trans fat per serving: 0 gm

Total fat per serving: 4 gms

Cauliflower Purée

Serves 4

Chef Michelle Bernstein
Miami, Florida

1 head of cauliflower,
  chopped
¼ cup low-fat milk

1 tsp lemon zest
¼ tsp ground nutmeg
Salt and pepper to taste

Place all ingredients in a large saucepan on medium heat. Cook until cauliflower is very soft. Strain well and place in a blender. Purée in blender.

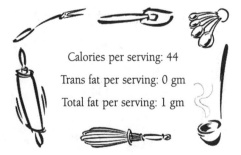

Calories per serving: 44
Trans fat per serving: 0 gm
Total fat per serving: 1 gm

Fast and Delicious Zucchini

Serves 8 to 10

Chef Michelle Bernstein
Miami, Florida

3 Tbsp olive oil
4 cloves garlic, crushed
6 medium zucchini, sliced in
   1/4 inch slices

2 medium onions, sliced thin
3 Tbsp fresh dill, chopped fine
Salt and pepper to taste

Place 1 tablespoon olive oil at the bottom of a skillet on low heat. Layer as follows: crushed garlic, double layer of zucchini, onions, dill, drizzle of oil, salt and pepper. Repeat this layer until all ingredients are gone. Cover and cook on low to medium heat until tender, about 20 minutes.

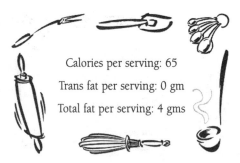

Calories per serving: 65

Trans fat per serving: 0 gm

Total fat per serving: 4 gms

Broccoli Souffle

Serves 4 to 6

2 (10 oz.) packages frozen
chopped broccoli
2 eggs plus 2 additional
egg whites
Salt and pepper to taste
1 Tbsp Campbell's onion soup mix

½ cup Hellmann's Light
mayonnaise
2 Tbsp flour
PAM cooking spray

Preheat oven to 350 degrees. Cook broccoli according to package directions. Drain thoroughly. Set aside. In a mixing bowl, beat the eggs and egg whites very well. Add salt, pepper and onion soup mix; add the mayonnaise and continue beating until well blended. Stir in the cooked broccoli. Spray a 7 x 11½ inch baking dish. Dust it lightly with 1 tablespoon flour. Pour in the broccoli mixture and sprinkle with the remaining flour. Bake for 40 to 50 minutes, until the top is golden brown.

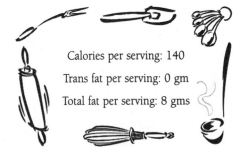

Calories per serving: 140
Trans fat per serving: 0 gm
Total fat per serving: 8 gms

Oven Roasted Vegetables

Serves 8

4 carrots	1 tsp dried rosemary
4 small red potatoes	1 tsp dried thyme
2 medium winter squash	³/₄ tsp salt *(optional)*
2 onions	¹/₄ tsp black pepper
¹/₄ cup olive oil	

Preheat oven to 425 degrees. Pare carrots and slice into sticks. Scrub potatoes; cut into quarters. Scrub squash and slice. Peel onions and slice into quarters. Combine vegetables except squash and toss with olive oil. Place in a casserole dish. Sprinkle with herbs and seasonings and bake for 20 minutes, covered. Add squash to casserole, stir and re-cover. Bake for 25 more minutes or until vegetables are tender.

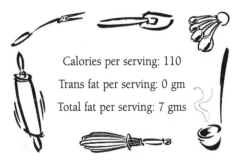

Calories per serving: 110

Trans fat per serving: 0 gm

Total fat per serving: 7 gms

The Carbohydrate Creations

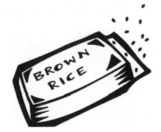

Colorful Potato Wedges

Serves 8 to 10

PAM cooking spray
3 medium sweet potatoes,
  cut into wedges
3 medium white potatoes,
  cut into wedges

1 Tbsp garlic powder
Salt and pepper to taste
2 Tbsp brown sugar

Preheat oven to 350 degrees. Spray PAM on a baking sheet. Place all potato wedges on baking sheet. Separate the white from the sweet potatoes. Sprinkle white potato wedges with garlic powder, salt and pepper. Sprinkle sweet potatoes with brown sugar. Spray cooking spray again on top of the potatoes. Bake 50 to 60 minutes, or until tender.

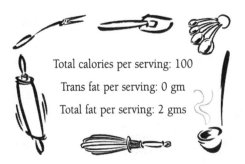

Total calories per serving: 100

Trans fat per serving: 0 gm

Total fat per serving: 2 gms

Very Vegetable Couscous

Serves 12 to 15

3 cups couscous, dry	¼ cup sun-dried tomatoes
3 Tbsp olive or canola oil	½ cup golden raisins
4 cloves garlic, minced	⅓ cup olives
3 scallions, chopped	⅓ cup balsamic vinegar

Cook couscous according to package directions. Sauté garlic, scallions and sun-dried tomatoes in olive or canola oil. Mix together couscous, garlic and scallion mixture. Add the raisins, olives and balsamic vinegar. Serve warm or at room temperature.

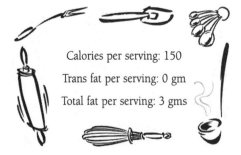

Calories per serving: 150

Trans fat per serving: 0 gm

Total fat per serving: 3 gms

Brown Rice Cakes

Serves 8

3 cups cooked brown rice
3 eggs plus 6 egg whites,
   slightly beaten
1 small onion, finely chopped
2 Tbsp fresh parsley,
   finely chopped

1 tomato finely chopped
2 Tbsp chives, minced
2 Tbsp thyme, minced
2 Tbsp olive oil

Combine brown rice, egg/egg whites, onion, parsley, tomato, chives and thyme. Mold into 8 to 12 cakes. Heat olive oil on low and pan-fry cakes until golden brown. Serve with low-fat sour cream and/or black beans.

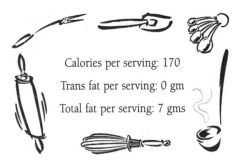

Calories per serving: 170

Trans fat per serving: 0 gm

Total fat per serving: 7 gms

Sweet Potato Soufflé

Serves 8 to 10

4 large sweet potatoes, peeled
and cut in quarters
²/₃ cup low-fat milk, scalded
2 tsp ground cinnamon
1 tsp ground nutmeg
PAM cooking spray

¹/₂ cup maple syrup or sugar-free
pancake syrup
²/₃ cup chopped pecans
1 cup rolled oats

Preheat oven to 400 degrees. Cook the sweet potatoes in a pot of boiling water until very tender. Drain and transfer to a large mixing bowl. Mash the sweet potatoes, milk, half the cinnamon and nutmeg. Spray a 13 x 9-inch casserole dish with cooking spray. Pour the sweet potato mixture into casserole dish and smooth with a spatula. In a small bowl, toss the remaining cinnamon and nutmeg with the pecans and oatmeal. Spread evenly over the potatoes. Bake for 35 to 40 minutes on top rack of oven, or until the topping appears a little brown and crispy.

Calories per serving: 160
Trans fat per serving: 0 gm
Total fat per serving: 5 gms

Creamy Corn Pudding

Serves 10

½ cup sugar
4 Tbsp corn starch
Salt and pepper to taste
2 cans creamed style corn
1 can corn niblets

3 eggs plus 4 egg whites,
   lightly beaten
½ cup low-fat milk
¼ cup Smart Balance margarine,
   melted
PAM cooking spray

Preheat oven to 400 degrees. In a small bowl, combine sugar, corn starch, salt and pepper. In a larger bowl, place creamed corn, corn niblets, and beaten eggs and mix well. Add dry ingredients and mix. Stir in milk and melted margarine. Place in casserole dish sprayed with cooking spray. Bake for 1 hour, stirring once.

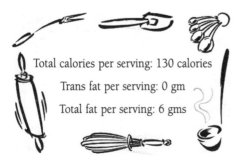

Total calories per serving: 130 calories

Trans fat per serving: 0 gm

Total fat per serving: 6 gms

Potatoes with Onions and Broth

Serves 6 to 8

2 Tbsp olive oil
2 onions, thinly sliced
4 large Yukon Gold potatoes,
  peeled and thinly sliced
Salt and pepper to taste

2 to 3 cups chicken broth
1/4 cup Kellogg's corn flake
  crumbs
3 Tbsp Parmesan cheese, grated

Heat the olive oil in a medium skillet *(that is oven-safe)*. Sauté the onions over medium heat, stirring frequently. Slice into quarter-inch pieces. Stir the potato slices into the onions and season with salt and pepper. Add enough broth to cover the potatoes and bring to a boil. Reduce heat and simmer 15 minutes or until tender. Press down and flatten the potatoes with a fork or spatula. Sprinkle with corn flake crumbs and Parmesan cheese. Place under the broiler until top is golden brown, approximately 1 minute. Watch it carefully!

Calories per serving: 115
Trans fat per serving: 0 gm
Total fat per serving: 4 gms

Whole Wheat Penne with White Bean Sauce

Serves 10

1 pound whole wheat penne
  or rigatoni
¼ cup olive oil
4 large garlic cloves, finely
  chopped
1 celery stalk, finely chopped
1 (19 ounce) can cannellini beans,
  drained

1 large tomato, chopped
1 tsp dried basil
¼ cup fresh parsley, chopped
Salt and pepper to taste
Parmesan cheese, grated
  (optional)

Bring a large pot of water to boil. Add pasta and cook until al dente. Heat olive oil in a large skillet. Add garlic and celery, cook until celery is tender, about 4 minutes. Add beans, tomato, basil, parsley, salt and pepper, and cook for about 5 minutes or until thickened. Drain the pasta. Toss the pasta with sauce and serve immediately. Offer Parmesan cheese.

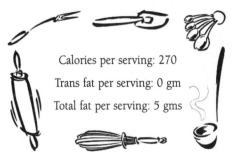

Calories per serving: 270

Trans fat per serving: 0 gm

Total fat per serving: 5 gms

Salads

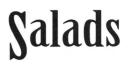

Mandarin and Peanut Salad

Serves 6 to 8

1 cup diced celery
1 head Romaine lettuce,
  chopped

1 small can mandarin oranges,
  drained
4 Tbsp honey roasted peanuts

DRESSING:
1 tsp dry mustard
3 Tbsp sugar
⅓ cup canola oil

2 Tbsp sesame oil
6 Tbsp rice wine vinegar

Mix celery and romaine lettuce together. Add oranges, peanuts and dressing right before serving.

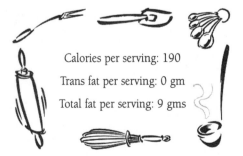

Calories per serving: 190

Trans fat per serving: 0 gm

Total fat per serving: 9 gms

READER/CUSTOMER CARE SURVEY

We care about your opinions! Please take a moment to fill out our online Reader Survey at **http://survey.hcibooks.com**. As a **"THANK YOU"** you will receive a **VALUABLE INSTANT COUPON** towards future book purchases as well as a **SPECIAL GIFT** available only online! Or, you may mail this card back to us and we will send you a copy of our exciting catalog with your valuable coupon inside.

(PLEASE PRINT IN ALL CAPS)

First Name _____ MI. _____ Last Name _____

Address _____ City _____

State _____ Zip _____ Email _____

1. Gender
- ❑ Female ❑ Male

2. Age
- ❑ 8 or younger ❑ 13-16
- ❑ 9-12 ❑ 17-20
- ❑ 17-20 ❑ 21-30
- ❑ 31+

3. Did you receive this book as a gift?
- ❑ Yes ❑ No

4. Annual Household Income
- ❑ under $25,000
- ❑ $25,000 - $34,999
- ❑ $35,000 - $49,999
- ❑ $50,000 - $74,999
- ❑ over $75,000

5. What are the ages of the children living in your house?
- ❑ 0 - 14 ❑ 15+

6. Marital Status
- ❑ Single
- ❑ Married
- ❑ Divorced
- ❑ Widowed

7. How did you find out about the book?
(please choose one)
- ❑ Recommendation
- ❑ Store Display
- ❑ Online
- ❑ Catalog/Mailing
- ❑ Interview/Review

8. Where do you usually buy books?
(please choose one)
- ❑ Bookstore
- ❑ Online
- ❑ Book Club/Mail Order
- ❑ Price Club (Sam's Club, Costco's, etc.)
- ❑ Retail Store (Target, Wal-Mart, etc.)

9. What subject do you enjoy reading about the most?
(please choose one)
- ❑ Parenting/Family
- ❑ Relationships
- ❑ Recovery/Addictions
- ❑ Health/Nutrition
- ❑ Christianity
- ❑ Spirituality/Inspiration
- ❑ Business Self-help
- ❑ Women's Issues
- ❑ Sports

10. What attracts you most to a book?
(please choose one)
- ❑ Title
- ❑ Cover Design
- ❑ Author
- ❑ Content

TAPE IN MIDDLE; DO NOT STAPLE

BUSINESS REPLY MAIL
FIRST-CLASS MAIL PERMIT NO 45 DEERFIELD BEACH, FL

POSTAGE WILL BE PAID BY ADDRESSEE

Health Communications, Inc.
3201 SW 15th Street
Deerfield Beach FL 33442-9875

|ııll,ııll,ıl,ıl,l,ıl,ıllll,lıl,ıl,lıılıl,l,lıl,l,l

FOLD HERE

Comments

Asparagus Salad

Serves 8 to 10

Chef Michelle Bernstein
Miami, Florida

2 pounds of fresh asparagus
1 cup water
1 large red onion, sliced
2 hard-boiled eggs

½ cup red wine vinegar
¼ cup olive oil
Salt and pepper to taste

Place water in a microwave-safe casserole dish. Place the asparagus in the water and cook in the microwave for 5 minutes, turn the asparagus, and then cook an additional 3 minutes. Drain the asparagus and set aside.

Chop onion very fine in a food processor. Add eggs and chop for just a few seconds. Set aside. Combine the vinegar, oil and spices, and add to the chopped egg and onion. Pour the dressing over the asparagus.

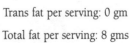

Calories per serving: 110
Trans fat per serving: 0 gm
Total fat per serving: 8 gms

Crab Salad with Gazpacho Vinaigrette

Serves 4

Chef Michelle Bernstein
Miami, Florida

FOR THE GAZPACHO:

8 overripe beefsteak tomatoes, peeled and chopped
1 bulb fennel, chopped
1 red pepper, seeded and chopped
1 cup Spanish onion, chopped

2 cloves garlic
1 cucumber, peeled and chopped
1 Tbsp chopped parsley
1 tsp salt
1 Tbsp sherry vinegar

Puree above ingredients. Keep refrigerated until ready to serve.

FOR THE CRAB SALAD:

6 ounces jumbo lump crabmeat
2 Tbsp lemon juice
1/4 tsp lemon zest
1 large Haas or Florida avocado, diced

1/4 cup cooked quinoa *(according to package directions)*
2 Tbsp extra virgin olive oil
1 cup diced cucumber

Combine salad ingredients. Plate the salad individually. For each serving, place a rounded scoop of crab-meat salad in the center of the plate. Pour the gazpacho vinaigrette around the salad.

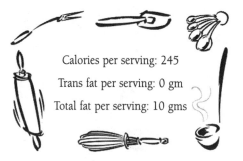

Calories per serving: 245

Trans fat per serving: 0 gm

Total fat per serving: 10 gms

Pear Walnut Gorgonzola Salad

Serves 8

6 Romaine lettuce leaves,
  chopped
1 medium pear, chopped
¹/₄ cup walnuts, chopped

¹/₄ cup dried cherries or
  cranberries
6 ounces gorgonzola cheese
¹/₂ medium onion, chopped finely

Chop vegetables and mix all ingredients together for a fresh, light taste.

DRESSING:

¹/₂ cup balsamic vinegar
3 Tbsp olive oil
2 Tbsp skim milk

2 tsp Dijon mustard
Salt and pepper to taste

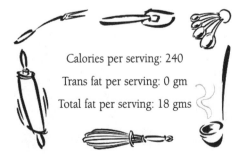

Calories per serving: 240
Trans fat per serving: 0 gm
Total fat per serving: 18 gms

Crispy Chinese Salad

Serves 6 to 8

1 large bag coleslaw
1 package Nissin Cup Noodles

4 scallions, chopped
½ cup sliced almonds

DRESSING:
6 Tbsp balsamic vinegar
¼ cup olive oil

2 Tbsp sugar
1 tsp pepper

Mix all salad ingredients together. Prepare dressing, add to salad and serve chilled.

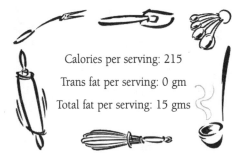

Calories per serving: 215
Trans fat per serving: 0 gm
Total fat per serving: 15 gms

Desserts

Strawberry Mousse

Serves 10 to 12

3 (3 oz.) packages strawberry sugar-free Jell-O	1 pint low-fat strawberry ice cream
2 cups water	1 pint low-fat sour cream

Add the 3 packages of Jell-O to 2 cups boiling water. Allow it to sit for 3 to 5 minutes. Mix in low-fat sour cream and low-fat ice cream. Refrigerate for 4 hours. Enjoy this refreshing treat.

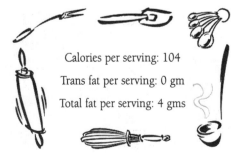

Calories per serving: 104

Trans fat per serving: 0 gm

Total fat per serving: 4 gms

Extraordinary Biscotti

Serves 18

Chef Michelle Bernstein
Miami, Florida

8 ounces almonds, pecans or walnuts, chopped	1 cup olive or canola oil
	2 tsp vanilla
PAM cooking spray	1 tsp baking powder
4 eggs	¼ tsp salt
2 cups sugar	4½ cups sifted flour

Preheat oven to 350 degrees. Toast nuts for 12 minutes. Set aside. Spray 2 large baking sheets with cooking spray. Cream eggs and sugar. Add oil and vanilla. Add baking powder, salt, flour and nuts. Mix thoroughly until dough does not stick to hands. Shape into 4 flattened loaves, then place on cookie sheets. Bake for 45 minutes. Remove from oven, slice on a diagonal. Place back on baking sheets as separate biscotti, and toast on each side for 5 additional minutes.

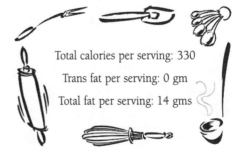

Total calories per serving: 330

Trans fat per serving: 0 gm

Total fat per serving: 14 gms

Banana Cake

Serves 12 to 15

¼ cup low-fat sour cream *or* low-fat plain yogurt
½ tsp baking soda
1 cup ripe bananas
¼ cup butter or Smart Balance margarine

1 cup plus 2 Tbsp sugar
2 eggs
1 tsp vanilla
¼ tsp salt
2 tsp baking powder
2 cups cake flour

Preheat oven to 350 degrees. Mix sour cream and baking soda. Let stand. Purée the bananas and set aside. Place butter (*or margarine*) plus the sugar in a bowl. Blend until creamy. Add eggs, one at a time, until well mixed. Next, add vanilla, sour cream mixture, salt and baking powder. Add bananas and continue to mix well. Last, add flour, slowly. Do not overmix. Place in an 8 x 12 greased Pyrex baking dish and bake for 30 to 35 minutes.

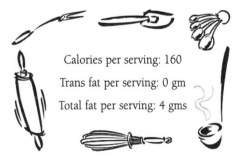

Calories per serving: 160

Trans fat per serving: 0 gm

Total fat per serving: 4 gms

Chocolate Brownies Light

Serves 16

PAM cooking spray   1 egg
2 ounces canola oil   ½ cup all purpose flour
1 cup sugar   Powdered sugar
½ cup cocoa powder
1 tsp vanilla extract

Preheat oven to 350 degrees. Spray 8-inch square baking pan with cooking spray. In a medium saucepan, heat oil over low heat. Add the sugar and stir until well blended. Remove from heat. Stir in cocoa and vanilla. Add beaten egg and stir. Stir in flour. Pour the batter into the pan. Bake for 25 minutes or until edges begin to pull away from the sides of the pan. Cool in pan on a wire rack. Sprinkle powdered sugar over the top. Cut into 16 squares.

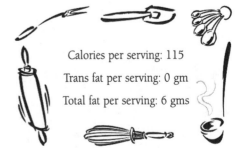

Calories per serving: 115
Trans fat per serving: 0 gm
Total fat per serving: 6 gms

Silky Tiramisu

Serves 8

1½ cups cold fat-free milk
8 ounce package light cream
  cheese, softened
3 Tbsp Kahlúa
4 ounce package sugar-free Jell-O
  vanilla pudding
1 tsp vanilla extract

2 cups Cool Whip Free, thawed
24 ladyfingers (Specialty Bakers),
  split
½ cup hot water
4 tsp instant coffee
½ tsp cocoa powder

Place ½ cup of the milk and the cream cheese in a blender or food processor (with the steel blade). Process until well blended. Slowly add the remaining cup of milk and liqueur. Blend in the pudding mix and the vanilla extract. Fold in the Cool Whip. Line the bottom and sides of 9-inch pie plate with 24 to 36 of the ladyfinger halves. Mix water and coffee and brush the coffee mixture onto the ladyfingers. Spoon half the pudding mixture over the ladyfingers. Top with remaining ladyfingers and repeat the process. Cover. Refrigerate 4 hours or overnight. Dust the top with cocoa before serving.

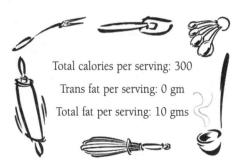

Total calories per serving: 300

Trans fat per serving: 0 gm

Total fat per serving: 10 gms

Peach and Berry Crisp

Serves 4 to 6

Courtesy of the *Miami Herald*

2 pounds ripe peaches
1 cup blackberries
1 cup raspberries

TOPPING:
3 Tbsp Smart Balance margarine
   (tub only), cut in chunks
½ cup brown sugar
⅔ cup flour

¼ cup sugar
3 Tbsp flour
PAM cooking spray

½ cup rolled oats
¼ tsp salt
½ tsp grated nutmeg
1 tsp ground cinnamon

Preheat oven to 375 degrees. Spray cooking spray in a 2-quart baking dish. To peel peaches, drop them into a pan of boiling water for 10 seconds, then put in a bowl of cold water. The skins should slip right off. Slice the peaches into a large bowl, in half-inch wedges. Add the berries, sugar, and flour and toss gently. Transfer fruit to the baking dish.

To make the topping, use your fingers and work the margarine in with the rest of the topping ingredients, to create a coarse crumbly mixture. Cover the fruit with this topping. Bake 45 minutes, or until the top is golden brown.

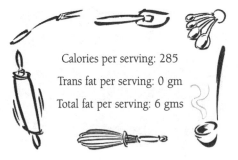

Calories per serving: 285

Trans fat per serving: 0 gm

Total fat per serving: 6 gms

Yogurt and Citrus Panna Cotta

Serves 8

Chef Michelle Bernstein
Miami, Florida

½ cups low-fat 2% milk
1 cup sugar
½ orange, zest peeled in strips,
    and juiced
½ lemon, zest peeled in strips,
    and juiced

¼ vanilla bean, split
4 sheets gelatin
¾ cup plain low-fat yogurt
1½ cups heavy cream,
    whipped

In a saucepan, heat the milk, sugar, zest (rinds), and vanilla bean, simmering until the sugar is dissolved. Meanwhile, place gelatin in enough cold water to submerge gelatin completely, about 1½ cups. Soak until softened. Once soft, remove gelatin from the water, squeezing out excess water. Add the gelatin to the hot liquid and stir until it melts. Let cool slightly, then stir in the yogurt. Strain the mixture into a clean bowl. Chill over an ice bath until it starts to thicken. Fold in the whipped cream. Pour into 8 individual 4-ounce molds or ramekins, or a large mold or ring mold. Chill for 2 hours. When ready to serve, dip in hot water for 10 seconds to remove the molds and turn them out onto dessert plates.

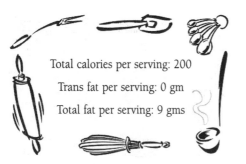

Total calories per serving: 200

Trans fat per serving: 0 gm

Total fat per serving: 9 gms

Magnificent Meringue Cookies

Serves 10 to 12

4 egg whites *(left at room temperature)*
1 tsp vanilla
$^1/_4$ tsp cream of tartar

$^3/_4$ cup sugar
$^1/_4$ cup Nestle semi-sweet chocolate mini-morsels
(optional)

Preheat oven to 225 degrees. Beat egg whites, immediately adding vanilla and cream of tartar. When egg whites become fluffy, slowly add sugar. Continue beating until stiff. Fold in chocolate chips if desired. Place by teaspoon onto cookie sheets lined with wax paper. Bake for 1½ hours. Turn off oven, leave meringues in the oven to cool.

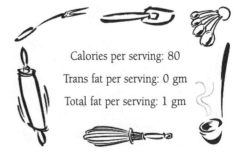

Calories per serving: 80
Trans fat per serving: 0 gm
Total fat per serving: 1 gm

Chocolate Amaretto Cheesecake

Serves 12

10 Nabisco chocolate-flavored
   ice cream cones, finely crushed
1½ cups low-fat cream cheese
1 cup sugar
1 cup 1% low-fat cottage cheese
¼ cup plus 2 Tbsp unsweetened
   cocoa

¼ cup all purpose flour
¼ cup Amaretto *(optional)*
1 tsp vanilla extract
1 egg
2 Tbsp semisweet chocolate
   mini-morsels

Preheat oven to 300 degrees. Sprinkle chocolate cone crumbs in bottom of a 7-inch springform pan. Set aside. In food processor (steel blade), add cream cheese, sugar, cottage cheese, cocoa, flour, Amaretto and vanilla. Blend until smooth. Add egg and process just until blended. Fold in the chocolate morsels.

Slowly pour the mixture over crumbs in the pan. Bake for 60 to 70 minutes or until cheesecake sets. Cool on wire rack. Cover and chill for at least 8 hours. Remove the sides of the pan and transfer to a serving platter.

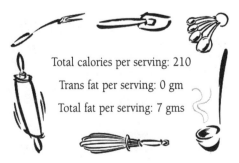

Total calories per serving: 210

Trans fat per serving: 0 gm

Total fat per serving: 7 gms

Fresh Strawberry Granita

Serves 10

1 cup hot water	3 cups sliced hulled strawberries,
¾ cup sugar	plus additional for garnish
2 Tbsp fresh lemon juice	

Stir first 3 ingredients together until sugar dissolves. Blend 3 cups strawberries in food processor until smooth. Add sugar syrup and blend until combined. Pour mixture into a nonstick metal baking pan (13 x 9). Freeze until icy around edges, about 25 minutes. Using a fork, stir icy portions to center of pan every 20 to 30 minutes for about 2 hours. Scrape granita into bowls and garnish with remaining berries.

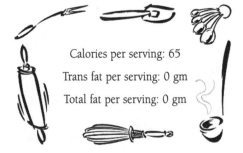

Calories per serving: 65

Trans fat per serving: 0 gm

Total fat per serving: 0 gm

Chocolate Peanut Butter Cookies

Serves 18

1 cup Skippy Natural peanut
  butter
½ cup sugar
1 egg

½ cup Nestle semisweet
  chocolate morsels
½ cup peanuts, chopped

Preheat oven to 325 degrees. Mix together peanut butter, sugar and egg. Blend until smooth. Refrigerate for ½ hour. Roll dough into 18 peanut butter balls. Place on ungreased baking sheet, about 2 inches apart, and flatten into cookie. Bake for 20 minutes or until lightly browned. In the meantime, melt chocolate morsels in microwave (about 1 to 2 minutes). Dip cooled cookies in chocolate, then in peanuts. Refrigerate until chocolate becomes hard.

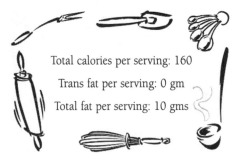

Total calories per serving: 160

Trans fat per serving: 0 gm

Total fat per serving: 10 gms

Brunch

Spinach Frittata

Serves 4 to 6

Chef Michelle Bernstein
Miami, Florida

12-ounce package fresh spinach
1 large onion
1 Tbsp olive oil
1 cup sliced mushrooms

½ cup Egg Beaters or 6 egg whites
Salt and pepper to taste
PAM cooking spray

Cut raw spinach in thin pieces. Slice onions thin and sauté spinach and onion in medium frying pan with olive oil. Use low heat and sauté until transparent. Beat egg whites/Egg Beaters in small bowl; add the onions, mushrooms, salt and pepper. Spray frying pan with cooking spray and return mixture to hot frying pan. Cook on low heat for about 15 minutes. Flip *(or put on a large plate, turn it over, and slide back into frying pan)* and finish cooking for 10 to 15 minutes on low heat. Serve warm or cold.

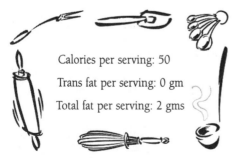

Calories per serving: 50

Trans fat per serving: 0 gm

Total fat per serving: 2 gms

Mango Bisque

Serves 4 to 6

3 mangos, peeled, seeded and
cubed
Juice of 1 to 2 limes
(taste after first lime)

1 cup plain nonfat Dannon
yogurt
1 cup skim or low-fat milk
Dash cinnamon and/or nutmeg

Place all ingredients in a food processor or blender and process
until smooth. Chill and serve this light and delicious bisque.

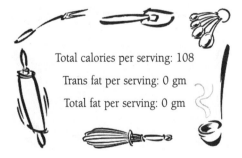

Total calories per serving: 108

Trans fat per serving: 0 gm

Total fat per serving: 0 gm

Stuffed French Toast Soufflé

Serves 10 to 12

2 (8 oz.) packages low-fat
  cream cheese
14 slices whole wheat bread
  (cut crust off)
PAM cooking spray
6 eggs

12 egg whites
2 cups low-fat milk
⅓ cup maple syrup
2 tsp vanilla extract
Cinnamon and sugar to taste
Powdered sugar to garnish

Cut cream cheese and bread into 1-inch cubes. Spray 13 x 9-inch pan with nonstick cooking spray. Spread cubes of cream cheese and bread around the pan. In a blender, mix eggs, egg whites, milk, vanilla and syrup. Pour over bread/cream cheese. Cover and refrigerate overnight. The next day, when ready to serve, preheat oven to 350 degrees. Sprinkle with cinnamon and sugar. Bake for 45 to 50 minutes. Before serving, sprinkle with powdered sugar.

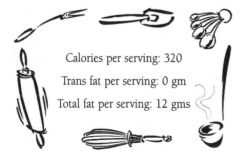

Calories per serving: 320
Trans fat per serving: 0 gm
Total fat per serving: 12 gms

Broccoli Quiche

Serves 6 to 8

4 Tbsp onions, diced
PAM cooking spray
1 (12 oz.) package chopped
  broccoli, cooked and drained
6 ounces low-fat Swiss cheese,
  cut into small pieces
3 ounces shredded or grated
  Parmesan cheese

3 ounces low-fat ricotta
  cheese
2 eggs
4 egg whites
1 cup 2% milk
Black pepper to taste

Preheat oven to 350 degrees. Sauté onions in cooking spray.
Mix all remaining ingredients together, and add onions. Spray
round baking dish with cooking spray. Bake for 30 minutes.

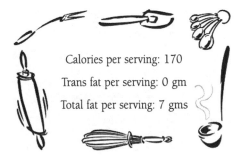

Calories per serving: 170

Trans fat per serving: 0 gm

Total fat per serving: 7 gms

Buckwheat Blinis with Poached Eggs & Fresh Lump Crabmeat

Serves 8

Chef Michelle Bernstein
Miami, Florida

BUCKWHEAT BLINIS:

²/₃ cup warm low-fat milk
½ tsp honey
1 packet dry yeast
2 Tbsp melted butter
½ cup plus 2 Tbsp all-purpose
   flour
¼ cup buckwheat flour
1 pinch salt
1 tsp baking powder
2 eggs, well beaten
1 Tbsp grapeseed oil

POACHED EGGS & CRABMEAT:

8 large eggs
½ tsp vinegar
1 cup low-fat sour cream
1 Tbsp lemon zest
1 Tbsp fresh dill
8 ounces fresh crabmeat
1 Tbsp lemon juice

For the blinis, combine milk, honey and yeast in a medium bowl. Stir until blended. Let mixture stand until foamy, about 10 minutes. Stir in cooled butter. In another medium bowl, combine flour, salt and baking powder. Make a well in the center and stir in milk mixture until blended. Slowly blend in the beaten eggs just until combined. Cover and let rise at room temperature for about 1 hour, or until the volume doubles.

(continued on next page)

Heat a skillet on medium high heat. Coat pan with grapeseed oil. Pour about 1 tablespoon batter into the pan and cook for 1 minute. The blini should be golden brown. Flip over and brown other side. Repeat with remaining batter.

For the eggs (*poached*), add vinegar and a pinch of salt to a large pot of boiling water. Reduce heat to simmer and begin stirring water clockwise. Crack the eggs, one at a time, into the water. They will take instant form. Cook for 3 minutes. Remove carefully with a slotted spoon.

To assemble: Combine the sour cream, lemon zest and dill. Combine the crabmeat with the lemon juice and season with a little salt and pepper. Place a blini down, put a poached egg on top, then top each egg with a tablespoon of sour cream mixture, then the crabmeat. Serve immediately.

Calories per serving: 300
Trans fat per serving: 0 gm
Total fat per serving: 14 gms

Potato and Artichoke Rosti

Serves 6 to 8

4 large baking potatoes	4 ounces shredded fontina or
¼ tsp salt	low-fat mozzarella cheese
¼ tsp black pepper	1 (8 oz.) jar marinated artichoke
2 Tbsp olive oil	hearts, rinsed, drained, sliced

Preheat oven to 400 degrees. Peel and coarsely shred potatoes. Pat dry with paper towels. In large bowl, toss potatoes with salt and pepper. In nonstick skillet (10 inches), heat a tablespoon of olive oil over medium heat. Add half the potatoes, gently patting with rubber spatula so potatoes cover bottom of skillet. Leaving a half-inch border, top potatoes with half the cheese, all the artichokes and then the remaining cheese. Cover with remaining potatoes, gently patting to edge of skillet. Cook 10 minutes or until browned, gently shaking skillet from time to time to keep pancake from sticking. Invert potato pancake onto large flat plate. Add tablespoon of olive oil to the skillet and slide pancake back into the skillet. Cook 10 minutes longer. Place skillet, uncovered, into oven and bake for 20 minutes until potatoes are tender.

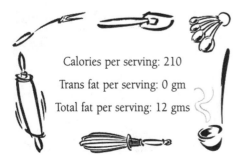

Calories per serving: 210

Trans fat per serving: 0 gm

Total fat per serving: 12 gms

Pasta with Broccoli and Beans

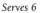

Serves 6

8 oz. whole wheat penne
  macaroni, dry
2 Tbsp pine nuts
1 red pepper, cut into strips
2 garlic cloves, minced
2 Tbsp olive oil
¼ tsp red-pepper flakes

1 large bunch broccoli, cut
  into small pieces
1 (10.5 oz.) can white beans,
  drained
½ tsp salt
½ cup shredded fresh basil leaves
¼ cup grated Parmesan cheese

Prepare penne pasta according to label directions. The remaining steps are prepared in a microwave oven: cook pine nuts on high 2 to 4 minutes until golden, stirring twice during the cooking. In 3-quart casserole dish, place red pepper strips, garlic, oil and red pepper flakes; cover and cook on high 3 to 4 minutes until pepper strips are tender-crisp. Stir in broccoli; cook, covered, on high 7 to 9 minutes until broccoli is tender. Stir halfway through cooking. Add the beans, cook again, covered, 1 to 2 minutes until the beans are hot. Add salt, then add the penne, basil and Parmesan cheese. Sprinkle with pine nuts.

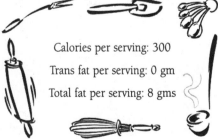

Calories per serving: 300

Trans fat per serving: 0 gm

Total fat per serving: 8 gms

Red Fruit Salad

Serves 10

Chef Martha Bernstein
Miami, Florida

2 quarts strawberries
2 pints raspberries
2 pints blackberries

2 pints pitted red cherries
2 lemons
6 packets of Splenda sweetener
Sprig of mint for garnish

Layer each fruit in a deep glass bowl, adding the juice of ½ lemon and 2 packets of Splenda between each layer. Cover and refrigerate for 1 hour until flavors blend together. Serve with a sprig of mint.

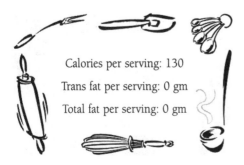

Calories per serving: 130

Trans fat per serving: 0 gm

Total fat per serving: 0 gm

Granny Smith Apple Pie

Serves 8 to 10

³/₄ cup Grape-Nuts cereal
Cinnamon to taste
1 to 2 cans Granny Smith frozen
apple juice concentrate

4 to 5 Granny Smith apples,
cored, peeled and sliced
1 Tbsp corn starch
¹/₂ cup water

Preheat oven to 350 degrees. Cover the bottom of an oven-safe pie plate with the Grape-Nuts cereal. Sprinkle with cinnamon, then pour half the apple juice *(thawed)* on top of cereal. Place sliced apples on top of crust, in circular form. Bake 35 minutes.

In a saucepan, mix the other half of the apple juice concentrate, corn starch and water. Cook on low heat until thickened. Pour mixture on top of apples after baking is complete. Refrigerate for one hour. Serve.

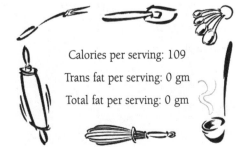

Calories per serving: 109
Trans fat per serving: 0 gm
Total fat per serving: 0 gm

Fresh Fruit and Ricotta Parfaits

Serves 6

1 cup low-fat ricotta cheese
⅓ cup sugar
2 Tbsp Amaretto liqueur
1¼ tsp vanilla extract
1 tsp unflavored gelatin
½ cup nonfat yogurt

2 large ripe peaches, peeled,
pitted and cut into ½-inch cubes
(toss with ½ tsp lemon juice)
1 cup fresh strawberries, sliced
¾ cup fresh blueberries

Combine ricotta cheese, sugar, 1 tablespoon Amaretto and vanilla in a blender. Blend until very smooth, about one minute. Refrigerate until chilled, at least one hour.

Mix remaining 1 tablespoon of Amaretto with 1 tablespoon of water and sprinkle in gelatin. Let stand for 5 minutes to soften. Then, heat this mixture over low heat, stirring until the gelatin dissolves. Place the gelatin mixture in a large mixing bowl and slowly whisk in the yogurt. Set the bowl into a larger bowl of ice water. Stir the mixture until it thickens to the consistency of egg whites and begins to gel, about 4 minutes. Immediately beat the mixture with an electric beater on high for 4 to 5 minutes until it is light and about tripled in volume. Whisk in the chilled ricotta mixture by hand.

(continued on next page)

Toss together the peaches and berries. Spoon a layer of ricotta cream into a parfait glass. Top with a layer of fruit. Repeat with remaining glasses. Serve immediately or refrigerate up to 2 hours.

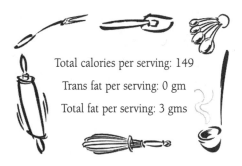

Total calories per serving: 149

Trans fat per serving: 0 gm

Total fat per serving: 3 gms

Crunch Top Blueberry Muffins

Serves 6

PAM cooking spray (optional)
2 cups all-purpose whole
  wheat flour
²/₃ cup sugar
1 Tbsp baking powder
¹/₂ tsp salt

¹/₂ tsp ground nutmeg
1¹/₂ cups blueberries
³/₄ cup low-fat milk
¹/₃ cup Smart Balance
1 egg plus 2 egg whites, beaten

CRUNCH TOPPING:

¹/₂ cup uncooked rolled oats
¹/₂ cup all-purpose whole
  wheat flour

¹/₄ cup packed brown sugar
1 tsp ground cinnamon
3 Tbsp Smart Balance, softened

Preheat oven to 400 degrees. Spray nonstick cooking spray into muffin pan (or use paper muffin cups) and prepare for 6 muffins. In a large bowl, combine flour, sugar, baking powder, salt and nutmeg. Add 1 tablespoon of the flour mixture to the blueberries, tossing to coat. In a small bowl, combine milk, margarine and eggs until blended. Stir into the flour mixture. Fold in blueberries. Spoon into muffin cups. Prepare crunch topping by combining all ingredients together until crumbly. Sprinkle the crunch topping onto the muffins. Bake 30 to 35 minutes.

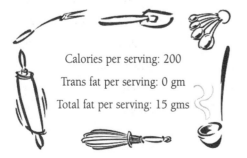

Calories per serving: 200

Trans fat per serving: 0 gm

Total fat per serving: 15 gms

Meal Planning for the Trans Fat Free Lifestyle

H ere lies the trans fat-free "meat and potatoes" of the Trans Fat Free Kitchen. Plan your meals around some of the following options, and your trans fat free lifestyle will be up and running! The chapter is segregated into children, teen and adult sample plans with one-week's worth of healthy interesting ideas for everyone to follow. It is not difficult to create this healthier lifestyle, especially if you keep to some structure and have available the trans fat free items you need for the week. Take it one day at a time, and I encourage you to set reasonable goals for yourself and your family. Remember to use Chapter 3 as your guide in the grocery store as you shop for your family and their healthier choices. Also, remember that the adult plans are *not* calorically based upon an individual's needs; therefore, use judgment in serving sizes.

Dying down, yet still important, is the carbohydrate craze, which has given us important information regarding the need for choosing healthier carbohydrates, that is, whole grains, whole grain cereals, white and sweet potatoes, beans, fruits and vegetables. The intake of refined carbohydrates is associated with heart disease as well.

We know it is a much better choice to eat whole wheat bread instead of white bread, brown rice in lieu of white rice and an orange instead of drinking large amounts of orange juice. These changes in our diets, as recent research has shown, may also decrease our heart disease risk, lower our triglycerides (these are cholesterol carriers in the blood), lower our risk for diabetes and insulin resistance, and hopefully limit obesity issues in this country, all of which have skyrocketed over the past decade.

TODDLERS AND SCHOOL-AGE CHILDREN (AGES 3 TO 11)

	MONDAY	TUESDAY	WEDNESDAY
BREAKFAST	½ cup Cheerios 4-8 ounces low fat milk small banana slices 4 ounces water	1 egg scrambled ½-1 slice whole wheat bread (Nature's Own) 4-8 ounces low fat milk ¼-½ cup fruit salad 4 ounces water	½ cup Quaker oatmeal 4-8 ounces low fat milk ¼-½ cup fresh berries 4 ounces water
LUNCH	2-3 slices turkey breast 2-4 whole grain crackers ¼ cup cooked broccoli ¼-½ cup blueberries 4-8 ounces low fat milk	1-2 low fat string cheeses 1 serving Goldfish pretzels ¼ cup green peas ½ sliced orange 4-8 ounces low fat milk	2-4 ounces grilled chicken strips ½ cup whole wheat pasta with tomato sauce ¼ cup green beans ¼ cup cantalope 4-8 ounces low fat milk
SNACK	Nabisco Vanilla Wafers	Low fat pudding	Orville Redenbacher mini popcorn cakes
DINNER	2-3 ounces baked fish sticks chopped tomato/cucumbers ⅓ cup mashed sweet potato ¼-½ cup fresh fruit salad 4-8 ounces low fat milk	2-3 ounces lean hamburger ¼ cup honeyed carrots baked french fries (5-10) ½ cup applesauce 4-8 ounces low fat milk	2-3 ounces tuna (low fat mayonnaise) ½-1 slice whole wheat bread 3-5 grape tomatoes ½-1 small sliced banana 4-8 ounces low fat milk
SNACK	4 oz. low fat yogurt	1 slice low fat cheese	Hot cocoa made with low fat milk

TODDLERS AND SCHOOL-AGE CHILDREN (AGES 3 TO 11)

	THURSDAY	FRIDAY	SATURDAY	SUNDAY
BREAKFAST	1 low fat Eggo whole grain waffle 2T Lite syrup 4-8 ounces low fat milk ½ sliced peach 4 ounces water	1 slice low fat cheese ½ Thomas' English muffin ½ sliced pear	4 ounces low fat yogurt ½ slice cinnamon toast (using Smart Balance margarine and ground cinnamon) 4-8 ounces low fat milk ½ sliced apple 4 ounces water	½ cup Quaker oatmeal 4-8 ounces low fat milk ½ cup applesauce 4 ounces water
LUNCH	1 T peanut butter 1 tsp jam 1 slice whole wheat bread ⅓ sliced cucumber ½ cup watermelon chunks 4-8 ounces low fat milk	2-3 slices lean salami rolls ½ cup brown rice ¼ cup cooked carrots ⅓ fresh mango 4-8 ounces low fat milk	⅓ cup low fat cottage cheese plus ⅓ cup alphabet-shaped pasta (mixed together) ¼ cup cooked carrots ½ sliced nectarine 4-8 ounces low fat milk	½ cup low fat macaroni and cheese ½ chopped tomato ½ cup lite canned peaches 4-8 ounces low fat milk
SNACK	Fresh fruit on a skewer	Low fat ice cream on a stick	Low fat granola bar	Vegetable soup and crackers
DINNER	1 chicken leg (skinless) ⅓ cup green beans ⅓ cup black beans ½ cup honeydew melon 4-8 ounces low fat milk	2-3 ounce lean steak ¼ cup green peas ⅓ cup rice 6-10 seedless grapes 4-8 oz low fat milk	1 slice homemade pizza (Boboli crust, tomato sauce and low fat mozzarella cheese) ½ cup lite canned pears 4-8 oz. low fat milk	2-3 oz baked chicken nuggets ¼ cup cooked broccoli ½ cup corn ¼ cup strawberries 4-8 oz. low fat milk
SNACK	2 Honey Maid Graham crackers 4 oz. low fat milk	4 oz. low fat yogurt	1 low fat string cheese	4 oz. low fat tapioca pudding

TEENS

	MONDAY	TUESDAY	WEDNESDAY
BREAKFAST	2 low fat Eggo whole grain waffles 8 oz. low fat yogurt 1 cup fresh blueberries 8 oz. water	1 cup Kashi cereal 8 oz. low fat milk small sized banana 8 oz. water	Grilled cheese sandwich: 2 slices low fat cheese 2 slices whole wheat bread (pan fried in PAM spray) small peach or pear 8 oz. low fat milk 8 oz. water
LUNCH	2 T Skippy Natural Peanut Butter 1 T all-fruit jam 2 slices whole grain bread baby carrots Baked Tortilla chips and salsa small pear 8 oz. water	3-4 oz. lean ham and low fat cheese sandwich Toufayan whole wheat pita lettuce/tomao 1 serving Baked Lay's chips fresh nectarine 8 oz. water	3-4 oz. tuna in water 1 T low fat Hellman's mayonnaise 6-8 oz whole grain crackers grape tomatoes 1 serving Genisoy soy crisps ½ cup melon chunks 8 oz. water
SNACK	Tortilla with low fat melted cheese	8 oz. low fat milk with sugar free Nesquick chocolatee Nabisco 100 calorie pack	8 oz. low fat yogurt 1 serving Nabisco Triscuits
DINNER	4-6oz. chicken on skewer ½-1 cup steamed broccoli ½-1 cup brown rice 15-20 grapes 8 oz. low fat milk 8 oz. water	4-6 pan-fried fish Chopped tomatoes ½-1 cup sweet green peas 1 cup fresh berries 8 oz. low fat milk 8 oz. water	4-6 oz. pork/veal loin Mixed Green Salad small baked potato fresh orange slices 8 oz. low fat milk 8 oz. water

TEENS

	THURSDAY	FRIDAY	SATURDAY	SUNDAY
BREAKFAST	1 cup cooked Quaker oatmeal 8 oz. low fat milk 1 cup fresh strawberries 8 oz. water	1 cup Honey Nut Cheerios 8 oz. low fat milk ½ cup fresh fruit salad 8 oz. water	2 scrambled eggs 2 slices whole wheat bread small sliced orange 8 oz. low fat milk 8 oz. water	2 slices French toast (whole wheat bread, low fat milk, 1 egg) 8 oz. low fat chocolate milk ½ fresh mango 8 oz. water
LUNCH	3-4 oz. turkey breast or turkey pastrami 2 slices whole wheat bread 1 T Hellman's low fat mayonnaise or mustard celery stalks 1 serving mini popcorn	3-4 oz. grilled chicken in a wrap chopped tomato/cucumber Low fat granola bar nectarine 8 oz. water	Homemade pizza with Boboli crust, low fat cheese, tomato sauce Romaine salad with Cardini's low fat Caesar dressing 15 cashews or almonds 15 grapes 8 oz. water	¼ barbequed chicken (skinless) 1 serving baked french fries cut-up raw vegetables 1 serving baked Doritos ½ cup melon chunks 8 oz. water
SNACK	8 oz. milkshake: 1 cup low fat milk, small banana, ice cubes, vanilla extract, Splenda	¾ cup Post Honey Bunches of Oats or General Mills Cheerios 8 oz. low fat milk	8 oz. low fat yogurt 1 cup sliced strawberries	½ low fat grilled cheese sandwich (Nature's Own whole wheat bread)
DINNER	Shrimp (10) stir-fry 1 cup mixed vegetables ½-1 cup whole wheat pasta ½-1 cup fresh fruit salad 8 oz. low fat milk 8 oz. water	4-6 oz. lean flank steak Sliced cucumbers/grape tomatoes ½-1 cup sweet potato wedges ½-1 cup watermelon chunks 8 oz. low fat milk 8 oz. water	Chicken fajitas (2) tomato, lettuce, salsa Corn or flour tortilla 15 fresh cherries 8 oz. low fat milk 8 oz. water	3-6 oz. tuna in water 1 T low fat Hellman's mayonnaise Toufayan wrap lettuce/tomato small sliced apple 8 oz. low fat milk 8 oz. water

ADULTS

	MONDAY	TUESDAY	WEDNESDAY
BREAKFAST	1 cup cooked Quaker oatmeal 8 oz. low fat milk small sliced banana 8-16 oz. water	2 scrambled eggs 2 slices Nature's Own whole grain bread with 2 tsp Smart Balance margarine 1 cup fresh raspberries 8-16 oz. water	1 cup Kashi cereal 8 oz. low fat milk small sliced peach 8-16 oz. water
LUNCH	Low fat tuna in whole wheat pita Lettuce/tomato 1 cup of vegetable or bean soup 8-16 oz. water	Grilled chicken wrap in whole grain tortilla Green salad with low fat dressing 8-16 oz. water	Goat cheese salad with olive oil and vinegar whole grain roll 8-16 oz. water
SNACK	2 low fat Bon Bell cheeses Nabisco Low fat Wheat Thins	15-20 nuts piece of fresh fruit	½ cup low fat cottage cheese 1 cup mixed berries
DINNER	Shrimp stir-fry with colored peppers and vegetables Large Mixed Green salad with low fat dressing 1 cup brown rice 1 cup watermelon 8-16 oz. water	Lean steak atop Large Romaine Salad with low fat vinaigrette dressing (Ken's) small whole grain roll ½ cup citrus sections 8-16 oz. water	Grilled tilapia fillet with oven roasted vegetables Large Field Green Salad with low fat dressing small sweet potato 4-5 dried plums 8-16 oz. water

ADULTS

	THURSDAY	FRIDAY	SATURDAY	SUNDAY
BREAKFAST	½ cup low fat cottage cheese Thomas' whole grain English muffin ¼ cantalope 8-16 oz. water	1 cup Uncle Sam's cereal 8 oz. low fat milk 1 cup fresh blueberries 8-16 oz. water	2 low fat Eggo whole grain waffles 2 T Lite syrup 8 oz. low fat yogurt ½ cup fresh melon chunks 8-16 oz. water	1 cup cooked Quaker oatmeal 8 oz. low fat milk 1 cup mixed berries 8-16 oz. water
LUNCH	Smoked salmon 2 slices pumpernickel toast Large Mixed Salad with low fat dressing 8-16 oz. water	Fresh turkey breast sandwich grilled vegetables 1 cup vegetable or lentil soup 8-16 oz. water	Egg white omelet with spinach, onions, and peppers Sliced tomatoes 2 slices rye bread 8-16 oz. water	Lean roast beef and low fat cheese sandwich with mustard (whole grain bread) small salad Individual bag of baked chips 8-16 oz. water
SNACK	2 T Natural Peanut Butter 3-4 whole grain crackers	15-20 nuts piece of fresh fruit	8 oz. low fat yogurt 2 c Smart Balance popcorn	15-20 nuts Dried apricots
DINNER	¼ skinless roasted chicken Sliced tomato and onion Steamed green beans with sliced almonds, 2 tsp olive oil 1 cup bean or lentil soup small fresh nectarine 8-16 oz. water	Glazed pork loin or veal chop Spinach salad with grape tomatoes, low fat salad dressing Ratatouille with tomato sauce small baked white potato sliced kiwi 8-16 oz. water	Grilled wild salmon Caesar salad with anchovies and Ken's Lite dressing Sautéed asparagus Couscous ½ grapefruit 8-16 oz. water	Ground turkey (breast) meatballs with tomato sauce Whole wheat pasta Cucumber and tomato salad small pear 8-16 oz. water

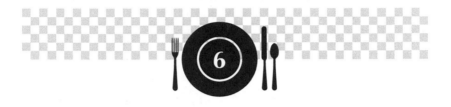

Trans Fat Free
Kids

For many children today, their healthy future doesn't appear very healthful and bright. It has been reported that our current generation of children could live shorter lives than their parents. President Bill Clinton, after his own heart and health issues, has partnered with the American Heart Association to bring this monumental problem to life. The Clinton/American Heart Association Creating a Healthier Generation Initiative kicked off in May 2005, hoping to bring to a halt the epidemic of childhood obesity in America.

The children in this country eat too much, make poor food decisions and move too little. It is our responsibility as parents to assist in the development of healthier eating habits from their first bite of food. We know how to teach safety to our children—do not run in the street, do not turn on the stove. We make sure they learn their ABCs. Why are we not teaching them the nutritional difference between eating a pretzel and eating a doughnut? Or baked potatoes versus french fries? How about teaching them how and when to indulge? Through the many years of counseling thousands of young children and their parents, I fail to understand this concept. Our children should be taught moderation in unhealthy eating, they should be taught when they are hungry and when they are satisfied, and they should be offered healthy choices and know how and when to make them. The goal is to create healthy independence with food.

Pizza, french fries and potato chips are among children's favorite foods, and their diets tend to be loaded with fat, including saturated fat and trans fats that are found in cookies, crackers and baked goodies. Children's diets also have too little calcium and fiber, setting them up for poor growth, and later, diseases such as osteoporosis, diabetes, and colon and breast cancer, as well as a long life of weight problems that will have its own horrific effects on their lives, both physical and emotional.

The following lunch and snack ideas incorporate a little less fat, more fiber, and are free of trans fat, which appears to be poison to children's arteries.

PACKING THE TRANS FAT FREE LUNCH BOX

The appropriate amounts of what your children need for their age group can be found in Chapter 5, *Meal Planning for the Trans Fat Free Lifestyle*. One trick toward teaching the healthy habit: pack just enough—not too much, not too little.

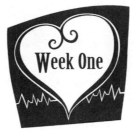

Monday:

❑ Peanut butter (Skippy or Jif Natural) and all-fruit jam sandwich (with Nature's Own whole grain bread)

❑ Small bag of baby carrots

❑ Nabisco "100-calorie pack" cookies or crackers

❑ 10 to 20 fresh grapes

❑ Bottle of water

Tuesday:

❑ Fresh low-fat turkey or ham wrap (Tumaros brand wrap)

❑ Small bag of baby grape tomatoes

❑ SnackWell's Fat Free Devil's Food Cookie Cakes

❑ Small peach or plum

❑ Bottle of water

Wednesday:

❑ 2 low-fat string cheeses

❑ Nabisco Reduced Fat Wheat Thins

❑ Celery stalks with natural peanut butter and raisins

❑ Hain Kidz Animal Crackers

❑ Small fruit salad

❑ Bottle of water

Thursday:

❏ Tuna sandwich (made with low-fat mayonnaise and Nature's Own whole grain bread)

❏ Smart Balance Popcorn or flavored popcorn cakes

❏ Chopped crunchy romaine leaves with sprinkles of Parmesan cheese

❏ Marie's low-fat or Naturally Fresh or Wish-Bone low-fat salad dressings (packed separately)

❏ Small sliced apple or orange

❏ Bottle of water

Friday:

❏ Beans and rice (may be served at room temperature)

❏ 1 low-fat string cheese stick

❏ Sliced cucumbers or pickles

❏ Pepperidge Farm Goldfish crackers

❏ Chunks of melon or pineapple

❏ Bottle of water

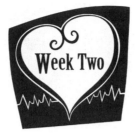

Monday:

❑ Grilled low-fat cheese sandwich

❑ Small baggie of pitted olives

❑ Individual bag of Baked Lay's chips

❑ ½ mango or small pear

❑ Bottle of water

Tuesday:

❑ Grilled chicken in a Toufayan whole grain pita or Thomas' Sahara whole wheat pita with lettuce and tomato

❑ Kellogg's Nutri-Grain Bar

❑ Individual container of applesauce (no sugar added)

❑ Bottle of water

Wednesday:

❑ Low-fat deli slices roll-ups

❑ Small container of whole wheat pasta with olive oil/Parmesan cheese

❑ Broccoli or cauliflower florets (with low-fat dressing to dip)

❑ Honey Maid low fat cinnamon graham crackers

❑ Small banana

❑ Bottle of water

Thursday:

❏ Skippy Natural peanut butter between 2 Eggo Nutri-Grain low-fat waffles

❏ Tomatoes and cucumbers

❏ Dannon low-fat Yogurt or Sprinklin's

❏ Small fruit salad

❏ Bottle of water

Friday:

❏ Roast beef in a Toufayan wrap

❏ Sliced pickles and/or baby carrots

❏ Quaker oatmeal squares cereal (small bag)

❏ Fresh grapes

❏ Bottle of water

FROM AFTER SCHOOL TO
SPORTING EVENTS

Include the following snacks in your children's after-school repertoire. As they begin to grow, remember to add trans fat free calcium choices to their snack times, such as:

- low-fat yogurt smoothies
- low-fat cheeses melted on a Thomas' English muffin (the muffin also has calcium)
- low-fat milk
- low-fat chocolate milk (make at home with trans fat free, low-fat, low-sugar syrups or powders, such as Ovaltine)

These and the following ideas will give them their greatest height potential. You may want to incorporate some of these fun and healthful trans fat free goodies, too.

- Yogurt smoothie (made with low-fat yogurt and fresh berries/banana/mango)
- Hummus and Toufayan pita
- Tumaro's flour tortilla or La Real corn tortillas and melted low-fat cheese (or soy cheese)
- Post or General Mills higher fiber cereal and a glass of milk (see the trans fat free treasures)
- Nabisco SnackWell's Fat Free Devil's Food cookies and a glass of sugar-free low-fat chocolate milk
- Angel food cake topped with Dannon low-fat strawberry yogurt and fresh strawberries

- Add a glass of milk to any of the following:

  Health Valley cookies or crackers

  Voortman's cookies

  Nabisco Kid Sense Fun Packs

  Nabisco Garden Herb Triscuits

  Thomas' whole grain English muffin with Smart Balance
    margarine and cinnamon

  Nuts and dried cranberries

Off to a baseball, hockey, football or basketball game? The best idea, of course, is to pack a hearty and trans fat free snack, as listed extensively in Chapter 3. You are safe with peanuts, (unless allergic) low-fat frozen yogurts and frozen lemonade. Question that soft pretzel, the popcorn, the pizza, the french fries and the cookies that you find at the concession stands. Hopefully, in the near future, trans fats will no longer jeopardize our healthy future.

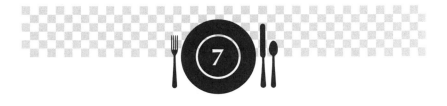

Dining Out
Trans Fat Free

We are busy people with busy families, most of us cooking a lot less than we used to. One out of every five meals in this country is served in a restaurant. So, as I sit with my clients and they confess that they are eating in fast food restaurants, Denny's, Roadhouse Grill and the Cheesecake Factory fairly often, I give them permission to have this hectic lifestyle *and* eat out. I certainly would rather we eat than skip our meals! I insist, however, that their fast-paced lifestyles can be healthy, low in fat, moderate in healthy carbohydrates, and trans fat free!

According to nutrition expert Dr. Walter Willett, Harvard University, "There now are alternatives that are available, and restaurants just need to take their customers' health to heart." Restaurants appear to be *slowly* coming around, painfully pulling themselves out of the trans fat quicksand, mainly changing the oil that is used to fry foods, such as french fries, fried foods and chicken nuggets. Partially hydrogenated oil has been used for all of these years because it has a long shelf-life, allowing the oil to sit for long periods of time waiting for fries and onion rings to enter the fryer. Once again, this has been shown to be torturous to our arteries.

I compiled a list of many restaurants, contacted each and every one of them, and asked for their cooking ingredients! Use this guide as you jump in for that quick bite, or, better still, when there is time to take a breather and enjoy your dining-out experience. These pages *do* suggest restaurants that either cook without trans fat or offer trans fat free healthier choices (through September 2005).

Generally speaking, when trying to choose healthier restaurant or fast foods, select items such as:

- grilled chicken or fish, or lean veal or steak
- whole grain breads, buns or rolls
- salads (dressings on the side) with or without chicken breast or fish or shrimp (can be grilled or blackened)
- baked white and sweet potatoes (watch the butter and sour cream—and eat the skin) or corn on the cob
- lean hamburgers (avoid the mayo and the cheese)
- wraps (preferably whole wheat wrap)
- low-fat deli sandwiches and subs (avoid the mayo and the cheese)

Feel free to ask your favorite restaurants what type of cooking oil is used. This quick question will make your heart smile back at you!

Au Bon Pain

Bagels

Cookies

Crème de Fleur

Muffins

Scones

Auntie Anne's Hand-Rolled Soft Pretzels

All pretzel doughs

Baskin-Robbins Ice Cream

All "Breeze" Beverages

All Cappucino Blasts

All "Creamy Bold Breeze" Beverages

All Ices

All Shakes

All Sherbets

Banana Nut Ice Cream

Berries 'n Banana No Sugar Added Low Fat Ice Cream

Black Walnut Ice Cream

Caramel Turtle No Sugar Added Low Fat Ice Cream

Chocolate Almond Ice Cream

Chocolate Chip Ice Cream

Chocolate Chip No Sugar Added Low Fat Ice Cream

Chocolate Chocolate Chip No Sugar Added Low Fat Ice Cream

Chocolate Fudge Ice Cream

Chocolate Ice Cream

Chocolate Ribbon Ice Cream

French Vanilla Ice Cream

German Chocolate Cake Ice Cream

Gold Medal Ribbon Ice Cream

Jamoca Almond Fudge Ice Cream

Jamoca Ice Cream

Mad About Chocolate No Sugar Added Low Fat Ice Cream

Maui Brownie Madness Low Fat Yogurt

Mint Chocolate Chip Ice Cream

Nonfat Soft Serve Yogurts

Nonfat Soft Serve Yogurts No Sugar Added

Nutty Coconut Ice Cream

Old Fashioned Butter Pecan Ice Cream

Peanut Butter 'n Chocolate Ice Cream

Perils of Praline Low Fat Yogurt

Pineapple Coconut No Sugar Added Low Fat Ice Cream

Pistachio Almond Ice Cream

Pralines 'n Cream

Raspberry Cheese Louise Low Fat Yogurt

Reese's Peanut Butter Cup Ice Cream

Rocky Road Ice Cream

Tin Roof Sundae No Sugar Added Low Fat Ice Cream

Vanilla Ice Cream

Vanilla Nonfat Yogurt

Very Berry Strawberry Ice Cream

Ben and Jerry's Ice Cream

All flavors

Blimpie

All cold cuts and cheeses

All salads and dressings

All sub rolls

Banana Nut Muffin

Blueberry Muffin

Bran & Raisin Muffin

Chicken Noodle Soup

Ciabatta Bread

Classic Chili with Beans

Grilled Chicken Strips

Meatballs with Sauce

Mediterranean flat bread

MexiMax

Tuna Salad

Vegi Max

Bruegger's Bagels

NOTE: *Some franchises may alter their cooking oils—you must inquire in each facility*

Burger King

BK Veggie Burger

Buns

Egg Omelet

Sauces, dressings and syrups

Scrambled Egg Patty

Carl's Jr.

Beef Patty and Bun

Beef Taco Filling

Black Beans

Bread, Sourdough

Chili

Chocolate Pudding

Corn Tortillas

Dressings

Raspberry Parfait

Rice

Salsa

Pork or Chicken Taquito

Turkey, Diced Cured

Vegetables, Chow Mein

Vegetables, Garden Ranch

Carvel Ice Cream

Black Raspberry Purée

Butterscotch Topping

Cherry Bonnet

Chocolate Crunch and Brown Bonnet Mixture

Chocolate Ice Cream

Chocolate No Fat Ice Cream

Strawberry Pre-Pak

Strawberry Purée

Vanilla and Chocolate Ice Cream

Vanilla Ice Cream

Vanilla Low Fat No Sugar Added Ice Cream

White Bonnet Ice Cream Coating

Dairy Queen

Chocolate Soft Serve

Vanilla Soft Serve

Dippin' Dots Ice Cream Products

Einstein Bros

100% Albacore Tuna Salad

Asiago Cheese Bagel
Asiago Chicken Caesar Salad
Black Forest Ham Sandwich
Bros Bistro Salad
Challah Roll Chicken Chipotle Salad
Ciabatta Bread
Chocolate Chip Bagel
Chopped Garlic Bagel
Chopped Onion Bagel
Cinnamon Raisin Swirl Bagel
Cranberry Bagel
Cream Cheeses
Dark Pumpernickel Bagel
Everything Bagel
Honey Whole Wheat Bagel
Jamaican Jerk Chicken Salad
Lahvash Bread
Lower Carb 9-Grain Bagel
Marble Rye Bagel
Naked Eggs
New York Lox and Bagel
Nutty Banana Bagel
Plain Bagel
Poppy Dip'd Bagel
Roasted Red Pepper and Pesto Bagel
Roasted Turkey on Artisan Wheat Sandwich
Salt Bagel
Sesame Dip'd Bagel
Spicy Nacho Bagel
Sun-Dried Tomato Bagel
Wild Blueberry Bagel

Fazoli's Restaurants

All food items are trans fat free except: Six-Layer Lasagna and
Lasagna with Broccoli, Twice Baked Lasagna, Baked Spaghetti
with Meatballs, Meatball Submarinos, and Four Cheese and
Tomato Panini

Hardee's

Bun, Plain 4 inch
Bun, Seeded and Slammer
Chili
Cole Slaw
Eggs
Grits
Ice Creams *(except Cookies and Cream and Chocolate Chip Cookie Dough)*
Milkshakes
Nonfat vanilla yogurt
Sauces: BBQ, Smokey BBQ, Honey Mustard, Ranch, Santa Fe, Tartar,
Texas Pete Hot Sauce
Sourdough Bread

Jack in the Box

All cheeses and processed meats
All dressings and sauces *(except cheese sauce and Frank's Red Hot
Buffalo Dipping Sauce)*
Asian Chicken Salad
Black Beans
Breakfast Jack
Buns and Rolls
Ciabatta Bread
Deli Trio Pannido

Double Fudge Cake
Greek Salad
Ham & Turkey Pannido
Meaty Breakfast Burrito with Salsa
Meaty Breakfast Burrito without Salsa
Pannido Bread
Pita Bread
Roasted Corn
Southwest Pita
Zesty Turkey Pannido

Jamba Juice
All smoothies and Juices

Papa Gino's
All pizzas
Classic Minestrone Soup
Hearty Chicken Noodle Soup
Salad dressings
Shrimp & Roasted Corn Bisque

Pizza Hut
All pizzas (except for Thin'n Crispy and "4 for All")
   and Full House Dough
Fresh Express Salad kit
Spaghetti with Marinara sauce

Quiznos
Buns, luncheon meats and vegetables

TCBY

All flavors except Cookies 'n Cream

Uno Chicago Grill

Caesar Side Salad

Chicken and Broccoli Fettucini

Chicken Basil Chili

Cooking oils

Flatbread Pizzas (All)

Cheese and Tomato Deep Dish Pizza

Chicago Classic Deep Dish Pizza

Farmer's Market Vegetable Deep Dish Pizza

Four Cheese Deep Dish Pizza

Numero Uno Deep Dish Pizza

Prima Pepperoni Deep Dish Pizza

Rattlesnake Pasta

Windy City Chili

Wendy's

Buns

Chili

Diced chicken

Frosty milkshake

Hamburger patty

Plain baked potato

World Wraps

All sauces and dressings

Fresh vegetables

Fresh meats

Spinach Tortilla

Conclusion—
One Heart, One Chance

As nutrition science continues, so does our quest for valuable and accurate information. It seems to constantly change—which food groups we should not consume, low carbohydrate plans, low-fat plans, high protein plans. It depends on the decade!

In essence, if we get good information and we are willing to follow it, it allows us to fight disease with our fork. The bottom line is that we all deserve to live an illness-free life, with great quality in it. Research has shown for many years that we are in large part responsible for this.

The latest studies indicate the imminent need for awareness of this newly recognized trans fat, or partially hydrogenated vegetable oils or shortening. There has been a shift in the last twenty-five years, from consuming fats of animal origin to fats from vegetable sources. Scientists are expecting us to have healthier hearts and arteries as we responsibly remove trans fats from our diet world. Though the food manufacturers are stepping up to the trans fat free plate, consistently removing the harmful fats from their products, the fast food and restaurant industries are not moving as briskly as they should.

Here are the important items to be aware of as you begin to remove yet another "challenge" food to your list:

- Evaluate your own eating patterns. Decide what changes you are willing to make in your life, and in that of your family's life.
- Eliminate trans fats from your diet. Read nutrition labels. Understanding them is more important than ever.
- Limit your intake of total fat, saturated fat and cholesterol, and subsequently, your trans fat intake should be minimal anyway.
- Maintain a normal healthy weight while being attentive to total calories.
- Choose plenty of fiber-rich whole grains, fruits, vegetables, beans and other legumes.
- Eat more fish.
- Include a variety of foods during your lifetime!
- Drink alcohol in moderation.
- Stay physically active, forever.

Best of luck in your trans fat free venture.

Appendix

WHAT *IS* GOING ON IN
MY BLOODSTREAM?

Studies dating back to the 1940s began to identify fat in our diets as a culprit in heart disease in men and women. Other significant risk factors included high blood pressure, smoking, inactivity, genetics and being overweight. To date these studies continue, and the risk factors remain serious indicators. The Framingham Heart Study, observing residents of Framingham, Massachusetts, for the past fifty years, is a remarkable ongoing research project that has investigated why heart disease has been such a vast and serious killer for so many years. Due to their results thus far, managing one's total cholesterol, HDL (good cholesterol), LDL (bad cholesterol) and a few other indicators, such as blood pressure, body weight, insulin levels and inflammation in the arteries, have been found to limit heart disease and stroke in a vital way.

CHOLESTEROL:
THE GOOD AND THE BAD

Studies show that cholesterol may begin building up in our arteries at the age of about six years old or so. Cholesterol, a waxy-like substance similar in appearance to melted candle wax, is a product of the breakdown of fat from foods we eat. Our liver produces cholesterol, too, because we need small amounts for proper functioning of the body. However, the normal liver produces all the cholesterol we need. The cholesterol that shows up in our bloodstream *in excess* is either coming from a family history, a medical problem or from our food supply, those choices we make.

Where does the cholesterol come from in our foods? It comes from animal products—beef, eggs, organ meats such as liver, dairy products, lard, poultry skin, fish, veal, pork and lamb. *Plant products do not contain cholesterol. They never have. They never will.* When the margarine label or the peanut butter jar you come across reads "no cholesterol," the cholesterol has *not* been removed from the margarine or the peanut butter, it never contained any. Beware, however, of those few plant *oils*—the palm, palm kernel, coconut and tropical oils—that *can* raise our cholesterol levels, unlike the other plant fats. These can be found on the ingredient label, too.

As you may know, cholesterol is not the only fat measured and observed in the bloodstream today. Other "pieces" of cholesterol measured are HDL, LDL, VLDL, cholesterol-to-HDL ratio, and so on. Imagine if we took one complete or total cholesterol molecule and threw it up against a wall, it would break into many "pieces." It is those "pieces" that have received much attention over the years, and in fact, may be more significant in the formation of heart disease than cholesterol levels themselves. One of these is LDL, or low-density lipoprotein, considered the lousy, or bad, cholesterol. LDL holds on to cholesterol molecules in the bloodstream, and keeps them circulating within our bloodstream. HDL or healthy or good cholesterol, are molecules that grab on to total cholesterol and excrete it out of our bodies.

Laboratory results, found in your medical chart, reveal your "blood lipids'" or blood fat levels—total cholesterol, HDL, LDL, the cholesterol ratios, C-reactive protein levels (measures inflammation) and homocysteine (amino acid as an indicator of heart health), to name a few. Ask your physician to review these with you each time you have blood tested. These are important numbers to understand, and you will know better why your diet and exercise patterns are crucial in this process of longevity and good health. *The consumption of trans fat exacerbates bad blood fat levels.*

Here are the items generally listed on a laboratory report (beyond your own personal information, such as date of birth and the time and date blood was collected):

1. *Name* of the blood test (e.g., total cholesterol)
2. The *level* found in your blood specimen (given in metric units as milligrams per deciliter or milliliter e.g., 200 mg/dL)
3. The *normal ranges* designated by current medical practices (e.g., cholesterol 125 to 200 mg/dL)

Here is the description of these lipid/fat levels you will find in your bloodstream, and the current acceptable normal ranges:

Cholesterol: Less than 200 mg/dL

HDL: Greater than 35 mg/dL (important to note that if this level is greater than 60 mg/dL, there is a "negative risk factor," meaning it is a benefit to your heart)

LDL: Less than 70 to 90 mg/dL

Cholesterol/LDL Ratio: Less than 2.8

Homocysteine: 6.1 to 17.0 mmol/L

C-Reactive Protein: Less than 0.8 mg/L

Apolipoprotein A-1: Less than 25 mg/dL

Clearly, if these numbers are elevated (with the exception of HDL), your risk for a heart attack or stroke is much greater. The intake of trans fats increases the LDLs (the bad cholesterol), decreases the HDLs (the good cholesterol), and changes how our cells function for the worse—not to mention that with the current research on insulin resistance and the recently-recognized metabolic syndrome, this increases your risk further.

Important to mention briefly, new findings over the past several years that may correlate to high-fat diets, heart disease and obesity include the medical issues of insulin resistance and metabolic syndrome. Though all fat consumption in the diet increases these potential risks, it is certainly less dangerous to our beating hearts if our trans fat consumption stays low.

In that vein, we should understand how insulin resistance and metabolic syndrome play their part in the disease of the heart. The pancreas is the organ in our body responsible for carbohydrate digestion and absorption. Insulin is a hormone that is secreted (or released) by the pancreas. It helps the body to break down and use carbohydrate, which turns into blood glucose, or blood sugar. Almost like a lock and key, insulin "unlocks" the ability of the glucose/sugar to go from the blood to our cells, providing energy (or energy that can be stored for later use). Insulin resistance occurs when the normal amount of insulin released by the pancreas is not able to "unlock" the process that moves the energy to our cells. To maintain a "normal" sugar level, the pancreas over-secretes insulin, the cells do not respond, and a high blood sugar level is created. This may lead to diabetes, or Type II diabetes, as it is more commonly known in the medical world. This insulin resistance usually is combined with obesity, physical inactivity, a high triglyceride level, and a low level of "good" cholesterol, or HDL. Therefore, this is a serious health problem affecting the entire cardiovascular and endocrine (metabolism) system—actually all of our body functions. Putting it simply, these issues affect the basic function of all our cells, the building-blocks of our bodies.

Metabolic syndrome, or Syndrome X, is a cluster of risk factors of heart disease also associated with this insulin resistance. The risk factors include: a high blood insulin level, a high triglyceride level, a high blood sugar level, high blood pressure, and a low level of "good" cholesterol. In this day and age, these are all critical medical markers you should be aware of.

So, arm yourself with all of this knowledge, understand how you may be able to control your lifestyle and destiny, and make your choices. In the meantime, make your life trans fat free.

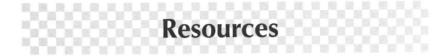
Resources

Y ou can find information regarding trans fats on the following
Web sites:

www.dietfacts.com

www.dietpower.com

www.3fatchicks.com

www.BDDiabetes.com

www.about.com

www.eatright.org

www.americanheartassociation.com

www.lipidsonline.org

www.cfsan.fda.gov

www.bantransfats.com

Notes

1 W. C. Willett and A. Ascherio, "Trans fatty acids: Are the effects only marginal?" *Am J Public Health* 84 (1994): 722–724.

2 W. C. Willett, et al., "Intake of Trans fatty acids and risk of coronary heart disease among women." *Lancet*; 341 (8845) (6 Mar. 1993): 581–5.

3 ["Fish and the heart." *Lancet* 2(8677) (30 Sep. 1989): 1450–2.

4 K. Oh, F. B. Hu, J. E. Manson, et al., "Dietary fat intake and risk of coronary heart disease in women: 20 years of follow-up of the Nurses' Health Study." *Am J Epidemiol* 161 (7) (1 Apr. 2005): 672–9.

NOTES

NOTES

Germ Freaks Unite!

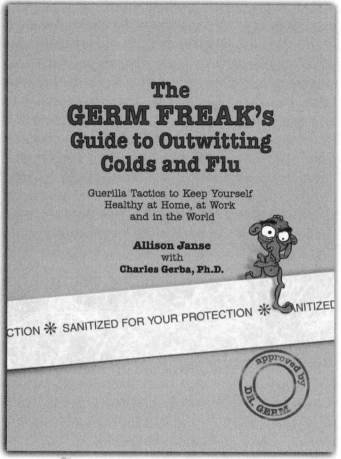

The
GERM FREAK's
Guide to Outwitting
Colds and Flu

Guerilla Tactics to Keep Yourself
Healthy at Home, at Work
and in the World

Allison Janse
with
Charles Gerba, Ph.D.

CTION ✳ SANITIZED FOR YOUR PROTECTION ✳ ANITIZED

approved by
D.R. GERM

Code #3277 • $11.95

This light-hearted but eminently practical book combines the knowledge of one of the world's top infectious disease experts with real world tactics of an everyday germ freak. Together, they give you straight answers on staying healthy with your sanity intact.
